Blueprint for Health

BLUEPRINT
for Health

by D. Stark Murray

SCHOCKEN BOOKS • NEW YORK

First SCHOCKEN edition 1974

Library of Congress Catalog Card No. 73-91343
Manufactured in the United States of America

Murray, David Stark, 1900—
Blueprint for Health.

Bibliography: p.
1. Medical care. 2. Medical care—Great Britain.
I. Title. [DNLM: 1. State medicine—Gt. Brit.
W275 FA1 M981b 1974]
RA411.M87 1974 362.1 73-91343

Foreword by Michael Harrington

It would be hard to imagine a more opportune time for the appearance of D. Stark Murray's book in the United States. It is now a quarter of a century since the defeat of the national health-insurance program proposed by Harry S. Truman; it is one decade since a part, but only a part, of the Truman measure became law in Medicare and Medicaid; and it is a period when conservative Republicans like Richard Nixon are finally recognizing that there has to be some form of health security for the American people.

But what kind of a program do we need? D. Stark Murray is ideally suited to help Americans answer that question. He is a British doctor who played a major role in effectuating the design of his country's national health system right after World War II. In addition he has traveled widely, studied health care around the world, and in this book presents an excellent summary analysis of various approaches to the problem around the globe. Finally, he has spent a good deal of time in America, lecturing and talking to trade unionists as well as other doctors. His insights are particularly relevant to our plight for that reason.

I will not even attempt to try to outline this wide-ranging study; it speaks eloquently for itself. Let me just preface it with a few comments about its special application to the United States.

First of all, America is, as Dr. Murray points out, utterly exceptional. It is one of the few nations on the face of the earth which still boasts—and boasts is, alas, the right word—a commercial, fee-for-service system. As a result, this country spends more on health care than European nations with national health systems, and yet its health is, as measured by objective indices, inferior to theirs. In recent years medicine has been one of the most important factors feeding inflation, not least because private health insurers have no motive to cut costs (and neither do doctors who reason that their fee comes from some independent source that can be overcharged at will).

But then these general statistics conceal the usual seamy side of American class structure. For those who suffer from the deficiencies of this extremely expensive and wasteful system are not the American people as a whole, but particular groups within the population: those of the poor under sixty-five not covered by an adequate Medicaid program (most states have pinch-penny programs); the aging who do not receive truly comprehensive coverage under Medicare (a group which President Nixon proposed to charge even more for their services in 1973); and perhaps most dramatically of all, the nonpoor working people who receive no government benefits and who do not belong to a union strong enough to negotiate a good medical-care plan through collective bargaining. I stress this last group for a reason. It is fairly well known that the poor and the aging suffer from inadequate health care. What is not understood is that the working men and women of America—and even a significant sector of the middle class—are also denied this basic right.

Second, there is now abundant evidence that the absence of health security for all actually encourages people to stay poor. In *The Politics of the Guaranteed Annual Income,* Daniel Patrick Moynihan, President Nixon's advisor on domestic policy from 1969 to 1971, described one of the most basic problems confronting policy planners today. He called it "the notch." Consider a poor family in a state with a relatively decent Medicaid program, say New York. In order to qualify for this health aid, its income must be below a certain point. Suppose that there is an upturn in the economy and it is suddenly possible for the head of the family to increase his or her income by $500 a year and thereby escape from poverty. However, that extra $500 of cash income might disqualify the family for Medicaid and lose them more than $500 in Medicaid assistance. They are therefore motivated to turn down advancement and to stay poor in order to get health care; or else they are forced to conceal the very existence of that income, lying to the government in order to keep body and soul together.

What is the answer to that problem? It would not even exist if there were comprehensive medical care for *all,* as Dr. Murray urges.

Third, and perhaps most immediately relevant to the present debate over health security in America, there is Dr. Murray's insistence upon preventive group practice. That idea is finally gaining acceptance in America. it has been endorsed by the Nixon Administration, which favors Health Maintenance Organizations (HMOs); a demonstration project has been funded; and the HMO is a central feature of the cost-cutting proposals in the Kennedy-Mills bill. The conservatives, like Nixon, still want to tie the HMOs into a system which relies on—and provides enormous Federal windfalls to—the private health-insurance industry. But the principle has at least triumphed. In Dr. Murray's book one discovers a wealth of practical data and experience on how best to implement it.

The book, in short, is of tremendous relevance to the America of the Seventies. D. Stark Murray is a practitioner in the best sense of the word: a man of medicine and of social conscience. He seeks not simply decent health care but decent health care within a democratically structured system where the people as well as the doctors will have a say. He knows Britain and Europe; he knows the United States. In *Blueprint for Health,* he makes a major contribution to an American health consciousness which, though decades late, is now becoming aware of one of the most intolerable aspects of our society.

New York City
March 1974

Introduction

All countries in Europe and North America now accept that the provision of medical care is a governmental responsibility, but differ in the method of provision and in the proportion of the population to be covered by any particular scheme. Most of the schemes have developed over a long period of time and so lack clear definition of the resources a nation can and should apply to the subject of health. In the United States, for example, a high proportion of medical care is provided by governmental agencies, by governmental subsidy and by insurance methods all 'concerned only with the rising cost of medical care and not with standards'. Professor Jerome Pollack of Harvard Medical School, from whom the quotation is taken, goes on to say that 'the mass purchase of care almost entirely without specifications is virtually without precedent in governmental action'.

Looking back on the development of the British National Health Service and surveying, by personal visit, the health services of twenty-two countries, it is clear that a great deal of what has been done in the United Kingdom and in all of those countries has been 'without specification', or on a specification that was incomplete, imprecise and often lacking in the necessary financial and other figures. It can be claimed that since each step in the development was in some sense experimental an exact specification was impossible; but it cannot be denied that an attempt to write one should have been made.

The author's attempt to write one for Britain, *Health for All* (Gollancz), in 1942, seemed reasonable in the light of the information then available; but it was partial and incomplete even for the UK and others of the same period had the same faults. It is surely time, with all the experience of the past twenty-five years behind us, to attempt a blueprint for the rest of this century, or at least to that year, 1984, which is so often used as a likely date for massive change. The present moment is also ripe for such an attempt for three very different reasons. First the policies suggested by the present Government in Britain would all produce changes in the organization of health services in the UK which must be seriously considered: for if the author's view that they are entirely wrong is correct, we must know what we should put in their place.

Secondly, the whole question of world-wide medical care is now being raised in many places as a result of two vast changes, the rapidity of transport and the increase in foreign travel, which means that more and more people may fall ill or have an accident causing injuries when away from home. This aspect will call for further study now that the European Economic Community has increased its membership to nine, for the Treaty of Rome will require all nine countries to have a considerable degree of similarity in the services they provide; and the movement of workers will involve reciprocal arrangements in the whole European area.

Thirdly, the position of the USA, and therefore of all its allies in NATO, is rapidly changing, and the need to provide health care for visiting tourists and workers on some kind of reciprocal basis will arise. Add this to the internal problems of health care, and it must be concluded that soon some form of provision, which both Democrats and Republicans have declared to be urgent, must be introduced. President Nixon, before his re-election, had already called on America to spend even more than it does in order to 'improve the delivery of health services . . . to provide more medical care resources in areas that have not been adequately served . . . and to encourage better preventive services.' But so far President Nixon does not appear to have in mind a clear specification of what is needed in practical terms, nor has he indicated how the specification, once ascertained, could be met.

The summary of the American situation on pages 45–47 is based on many years' study, but even since this was completed changes have taken place. The amount of money being spent is already nearly eight per cent of the G.N.P., and at the same time some projects have been cut in budgetary efforts to deal with inflation. The description of Medicare and Medicaid is probably sufficient for a general understanding, though changes being made at the end of 1973 have not been mentioned. They do not affect the overall picture.

In the delivery of health care the European system is ahead of anything that has been suggested in the US, and the British National Health Service is more soundly based and more comprehensively developed than those it may join in the Common Market. Nevertheless it has weaknesses and deficiencies and does not entirely meet the paramount need of medical science, the ability to absorb and use new methods and discoveries as rapidly as possible. Since health is indivisible and since the United Nations Declaration of Human Rights has established the right of all citizens of the world to health care, it would appear worth while to try to prepare a blueprint which will satisfy all these varied needs and demands and others that will arise as that task proceeds.

D. Stark Murray

January 1974

Contents

Tables

Figures

Chapter 1

Why we need a Blueprint for Health

Medical care as it has developed over the centuries, but with increasing speed and complexity in the past fifty years, consists of two related parts. There is the skill and knowledge of the individual doctor, extended in modern times by new skills and new types of knowledge of many other health workers and scientists, and there is the system of delivery of health care which at any moment depends on a combination of economic and political considerations. The skills are those of the trained individual who at all times has to take those responsibilities which his or her position dictates; the system of health care delivery rests upon the political and ethical attitudes of the society in which the health worker functions. Ideally as society develops and new concepts of how communities should be governed arise, the health worker should be in the vanguard, guiding the process and indicating how medical science can best be used for the greatest good of the individual and of the nation.

Three factors in particular have influenced thinking in this field. The first is the almost universal recognition that if health is a human right it must be someone's duty to provide a system of health care; and that someone is clearly the government or a governmental agency. Since government represents all the people this right must extend to every citizen, that is to say, the system must be one that is universally available. Universality does not dictate any particular form of care but it involves many other matters that have to be decided. Since a service for every citizen in a country will involve the recognition of many diseases, and discover many problems that have social and environmental facets, the service must also be comprehensive, and its aim must be to ensure that no one fails to get the necessary care however rare or unusual his health problem is.

The second, and related factor, is that no individual doctor can give that kind of comprehensive service but must have the assistance of and work with and through a suitable army of other health workers, the health care team. That team today spills over into social welfare, and no scientific form of health care and medical treatment can ignore any of the environmental factors with which modern man has to contend. In Britain this century began with the individual doctor working very much as a single-handed practitioner; today the British health team is one of the largest among the many forms of co-operative effort that exist. The health care team is also a great user of physical resources, and as technology continues to develop, the machines that aid the doctor, in diagnosis and in treatment, become more accurate, capable of an almost infinite variety of tests and examination, and become in the process exceedingly costly.

This is the third factor that has influenced thinking in many countries, the rising cost of medical care and rapid growth in the use of expensive equipment. As we shall see in later chapters, health now absorbs a moderately large proportion of any nation's total resources both in money and in workers. In the early writings on the subject in this country it was assumed that two factors would prevent costs rising too rapidly, if at all. It was thought that by using all possible preventive methods not only would lives be saved but fewer cases would have to be treated expensively; and that an organized service would use its resources much more efficiently and therefore more economically. Estimates made during World War II for a post-war service ranged between £140 and £190 million a year and a Labour Party document said that even if the latter figure was exceeded, 'the burden would still be a light one, having regard to the importance of the need and the size of the national income'.

Since then the cost of medical care has steadily grown in every country but the causes are complex and many are unconnected with health. Inflation and revaluations of currencies coupled with rising standards of living have altered every figure. An indication of the kind of increase in every country is given by the average weekly cost of a hospital bed in Britain, approximately (£30) $75, in 1962, and (£67) $170 in 1970. A large part of the increase has been due to new medical discoveries and above all to looking after people much later in life, who are subject to the infirmities of old age. These infirmities, sometimes hardly definable as disease, add considerably to the cost of a service universally available. This was, and is, one of the factors greatly influencing thinking in the USA, for the introduction of Medicare for the aged highlighted the amount of uncared for disease and infirmity which existed. Indeed the full effect of this has not yet been felt, for not only is expectation of life in American lower than in many European countries but the Medicare system is not fully comprehensive.

The escalation of cost has, of course, been greatest in the USA because medical costs there are still being met by market-place methods, by direct personal payments and by payments through third parties, the nation, state or the county, by insurers, whether profit-making or mutual, and by many other devices. In most other countries costs have been restrained, usually by forecast budgeting but when necessary by agreement between government as the main purchaser and the medical profession as the chief provider of care. In those countries which have retained 'fee-for-service' payments agreement has usually been sought and reached with the medical profession and is subject to regular review in the light of each nation's economic position. In America the medical profession has resisted all efforts to control the fees a doctor may charge, and these have risen continuously; and the system of insuring for hospital costs has led to some fantastic increases.

The trouble has been that it is only in an organized service that any attempt can seriously be made to control costs and relate them, which is more important even than control, to the service given. American experience in the last twenty years has shown that neither private practice nor insurance methods can either meet the need for a universal comprehensive service or control the cost of what service is provided. Private practice by its very nature cannot control prices or plan services: it is individualistic, competitive and divisory whereas modern medical team work must be co-operative and unifying. The ethical implications of this change are discussed later but meantime it must be emphasized that even the valiant efforts of the Blue Cross plans to pay for hospital care have failed either to restrain prices or to produce any unifying force. So there is no planning of the resources and the insurer and insured are both in the power of the medical profession which spends money on increased and improved resources without reference to those who have to pay.

As a result the individual can no longer pay directly for every form of health care. If he is wealthy enough it is just possible he might be able to pay for an insurance policy that would cover every contingency, but very few can do this. Nor do insurance people like to be asked to quote for every contingency, and in all countries where insurance still plays a part in medical finance insurance policies and programmes contain exceptions, diseases that cannot be treated, age groups that are excluded, procedures (especially lengthy ones) that are not paid for and so on. It is only when an nation has decided the care must be comprehensive that exceptions and co-payments can be ended.

When that decision is reached the system for the delivery of health care has still to decide how comprehensive the service is, for a poor nation could make the decision as a goal, as India has, without being financially able at this time to realize the aim. It must also be remembered that as no country has got a completely adequate comprehensive service and as medical science must go on and make new discoveries, systems must be capable of expansion. A new form of treatment, for example a real cure for cancer, might be very expensive in money, resources and manpower, but no service could be considered comprehensive if it did not contain the machinery for teaching and applying such a new treatment. At all times there are bound to be new, but impressive, ideas that must be tried out and a nation which cares for its health must be prepared to spend more when the need is clear; and the health worker team must be called upon to make conscious decisions as to priorities. That this will involve a greater sense of social responsibility in all health workers is recognized; how it is to be inculcated and how it is to work is part of the specification we propose to examine.

The list of things to be done is formidable; the ways in which different countries have tackled them is long and often incomplete. Historically there has been a common thread running through health care systems throughout the world. There has for centuries been a need for organized schemes at least for those diseases most dangerous to the community and those groups, the impoverished and disabled, for whom provision had to be made. It is said that in Greece in 600 BC it was already seen to be necessary to appoint 'community physicians' to cover areas and populations not otherwise served by medical men: and in Britain from the days of Elizabeth I the existence of the poor-houses with their growing and developed hospital sections was part of the growing proof, emphasized by the impact of the industrial revolution, that health care had to be an essential part of the services provided by public bodies. When the Webbs wrote in 1908 that Britain would never be healthy until it had a form of State medical service they were echoing what was being said in all European countries, and Britain's first big experiment, the Lloyd George National Health Insurance Act of 1911, was one part of a growing system throughout Europe. All countries had found they had to provide some medical care for all of their people and for many of them had to provide all the treatments they required.

The great bulk of what was provided was on an ad hoc basis. A need was recognized, a particular disease was seen to be a danger to the community, a group was identified, for example, the mentally sick, as unable to provide for themselves and so on. For all these groups new agencies were developed, by the local community, by the State, by the Church as charity, until there was in all countries a plethora of agencies dealing with health. This process has gone on longest and most intensely in the US and goes on there today: in most other countries the acceptance that care must be comprehensive led to a unification of services and to greater efforts to plan health care as a single service. This only recognized what we have already said, that health being indivisible and a problem both for the individual and for the State, the system that provides care cannot be split up among different agencies but must be unified.

This recognition was slow to come in even the most advanced countries. Services continued to expand, new ones continued to develop in haphazard fashion and there was no specification for even the individual parts and none for any of the more developed services. The Scandinavian countries, particularly Norway, came nearest to setting down what was needed to fulfil universal needs until between 1940 and 1950 attempts were made in Britain, by a great variety of bodies, to prepare plans that would be feasible, economical and yet comprehensive, scientific and ethical. In the period between 1920 and 1940 discussions became more and more political but from 1934 onward the provision of a universal service was on the programme of the Labour Party and the Conservative Party produced its own schemes, which were less comprehensive and still divisory. But the attitude of the British people as a whole was summed up by Sir William (later Lord) Beveridge in his report (1942), on *Social Insurance and Allied Services* in which he made his Assumption B that in any post-war social insurance plan there would be established 'comprehensive health and rehabilitation services for prevention and care of disease and restoration of capacity for work, available to all members of the community'.

That was a statement of principles rather than a blueprint. The Labour Party later elaborated this in a document declaring that the medical service must be planned as a whole, must be preventive as well as curative and must be complete and open to all 'so that poverty shall be no bar to health'. The document went on to outline how these points could be met technically, administratively and financially, but so great was the task to be done that the National Health Service Act (1946) was little more than an Act enabling the Minister of Health, and the bodies he set up to do the work, to begin working out the details of the service. We may find that this has still to be the way in a democratically controlled but growing service, and a new specification may always be incomplete because of new discoveries, but twenty-five years after the start of Britain's NHS an attempt to look into the future should crystallize British views and may be of help to those countries whose system of health care still lags behind the best.

Chapter 2

What is Health?

Health care, the reader will have noticed, is used here in the widest possible sense, very different from medical care and implying much more than the treatment of disease. But what is health and why does it need care? And why does it need that care on the modern scale in which a country spends between 4 and 7 per cent of its annual gross national product on it? In ordinary language people feel healthy when they are able to carry out all the demands of life, of work and leisure without need to think of their bodily condition. The World Health Organization charter translates this as 'a state of complete, physical, mental and social well-being and not merely the absence of disease or infirmity'. The inclusion of social well-being as a criterion of health may seem to some to be utopian but it is nevertheless a very necessary consideration, particularly in our urban and polluted environments. René Dubos in *Man, Medicine and Environment* (1968) prefers to regard health not as involving the complete elimination of disease 'but as a modus vivendi enabling imperfect men to achieve a rewarding and not too painful existence while they cope with an imperfect world'.

But imperfect man is an exceedingly variable creature with a great variety of physical and mental needs and, according to how he works, where he lives and what standard of nutrituion he reaches, requiring a great variety of assistance to achieve a state of well-being which he will recognize as such. To recognize a state of complete well-being is nearly as rare as to achieve it, for man's imperfect use of his environment, his imperfect use of his own body and his imperfect resistance to many diseases all conspire to keep many people below their optimum condition.

But if we ask what is the optimum state of health for the average individual living in good physical conditions, we are still unable to define it very clearly. Is freedom from disease to be the main criterion? If so, then from the start we may be defeated by the myriad of defects, genetic and inborn or incidental to pre-natal development, with which so many are born. Is it freedom from those diseases which man has proved to be biological in nature, and to which, by the use of vaccines, defences in the body can be alerted? If so, is that man healthier who has never met and has not had to resist these infections than the man whose blood has been artifically stimulated to resist them? Does health lead to a longer life and if so do we know how long a man or woman should live? Is the medically protected life which so many aged people now live really that state of well-being we seek to lay down as desirable? Is the fact that people enjoy life a sufficient criterion? Everyone knows the stories of cripples and otherwise disabled people who clearly enjoy life in spite of the problems which arise from their lack of conventional health. Are we to consider the contribution people make to the community, even if it is only by example, sufficient reason for regarding their condition as 'healthy' in the widest sense even if their care is a very expensive business? If we have gone so far what attitude can the community or the physician take about those born with terrible but non-killing defects? Is their misery to be taken as sufficient reason for withdrawing the medical and nursing care they get today?

Faced with these dilemmas, the answer both society and the doctors have given so far is that where there is life our scientific knowledge and technical ability must be used to protect that life. Society may however change its attitude and finally recognize that there are some conditions, at both ends of the life cycle, which are so far from any concept of health, and in which there is not even a capacity for pleasure, that medical care should be withdrawn. But society must not be tempted to reach this decision simply because the cost of protecting these marred lives is high. The modern affluent society should be able to find the resources for such care, and indeed will probably have greater difficulty in finding people to look after these cases, than in finding the money and physical resources necessary. Certainly in those cases where disability has not robbed the individual of the capacity to enjoy life and contribute to the lives of others, society's duty is clear. As Karl Evang, Norway's great health care pioneer, has put it: 'No disease is strictly a private and personal affair: its effects spread like rings in water. . . . A medical care system must be constructed so that all may benefit from it.'

When we speak of health care we are therefore indicating that not only must all benefit from the system but it must cover the tasks of identifying health and all departures from it. Health care must in the first place work at preventing those departures, and when that is impossible must develop methods of returning things to normal, or, as so often happens, indicating and supervising the extent to which the sufferer has to make compromises with his disability. At no point should the health worker, or the system of health care, be asked to justify what is spent in terms of lives saved or damage repaired, and a health care system must not be expected to prepare accounts like an industrial plant. One cannot measure the health of the nation or of an individual in such material ways.

There are, of course, some yardsticks which can be used as a measure of the overall effect of health care, and international comparison of disease statistics, or geographical comparison within a nation, may reveal ways in which the money spent on health care could be used to greater advantage. There is a conflict over priorities in every growing service and the doctor is no more exempt from remembering the cost of what he does than are workers in any industry. Both points will be touched on as we discuss different subjects but meantime we may ask whether medical science has over all had an effect on the individual and on society, and we must define what we mean by medical care. We have spoken of preventing disease, of curing illness, of restoring function, but do we do these by a unified and recognized system?

To the first question any examination of the condition of people in a modern society, any study of the health of school-children, of the hosts of infant and maternal mortalities, of the expectation of life, will show what changes there have been in the past fifty years. No one can attribute all the improvements to medical care, for social changes have been going on at the same time; but there are many specific instances in which new medical techniques have saved tens of thousands of lives. This applies especially to the infections which once caused large numbers of deaths and are now almost unknown in the developed countries. Diphtheria is a typical case. In Britain it was once responsible for thousands of deaths every year, but it is now almost unseen by UK doctors. The increase in the expectation of life, which has risen at least twenty years in this century, is to a considerable extent due to the prevention of death from acute infections, and this happens among both the young and the old.

But some statistics show the overall improvement medical science plus social change have made and at the same time bring out those places which lag behind the general average. One of the statistical tables which shows this up and has shocked Americans is that for maternal mortality, in which the rate per 100,000 live births is taken. All these countries, and most others, have greatly improved their figures in those 13–15 years but the US has lost its place in relation to the others and still has a very high rate. (Great Britain is far from

Table 2.1 Maternal Mortality in Some Countries

	1951–3	1966
United States	67.7	29.1
Sweden	69.0	11.3
Denmark	75.4	19.2
Norway	81.5	25.4
Ireland	143.9	28.9

the best, 21.0 in 1969.) The infant mortality rate reflects both medical and social factors. In 1968 Norway lost 12.8 infants per 1,000 live births, the UK lost 18.3 and the US 21.7. The absence of a health care system undoubtedly affects the US figures but probably not as much as does race. In 1967 the rate for white infants averaged 19.7, for non-white, 35.9. It is the same social factor, poverty, which pushes up the rate among black infants, for the poor get neither the nutrition nor the medical care they need.

While advances of a dramatic nature have been made in treating microbial infections, advances in some other fields have also led to the saving and prolongation of life in such widely different conditions as diabetes and pernicious anaemia. The great killing diseases remain those of the cardiovascular conditions and cancer in all its forms. In both of these the advances that have been made by better medical care and new drugs are somewhat offset by the fact that such treatment has carried more people into those age groups at which heart disease and cancer are most common. And while medical science has greater power to save life it is unable, especially in heart disease, to return many saved cases to full or even useful life. Here again man produces his own dilemma. He saves life, improves the heart with artificial aids or even transplants a new heart: and is left with a patient who is going to continue to need a great deal of expensive care.

Clearly medical care has two aspects, the development of the best techniques for diagnosis and treatment and, if all citizens have a right to medical care, a guarantee of the highest standard to every citizen. Cost is then largely irrelevant to the physician but society has a right to set out the terms and conditions within which the physician must work. One thing that is increasingly felt, and shown in the practical schemes that exist in different countries, is that in return for being able to prescribe everything he considers necessary for his individual patients the physician must no longer be paid by market-place methods. He must be given the best possible conditions in which to do his work and must never have to think of the financial or social position of the patient.

Society will also expect to have some say in the type of medical care that is being given. There must, of course, be safeguards for the individual against possible wrong, dangerous or negligent treatment, but there is also the wider question of the professional attitudes of doctors and of the education they have been given. Most countries have over the centuries developed a system of medicine generally classified as 'allopathic', although many of the remedies and methods used do not strictly fit the dictionary definition of that word—treatment by things having an opposite effect to the disease. Whatever the definition medical schools all over the world teach the same body of basic knowledge about anatomy and physiology and use very largely the same treatments. In recent years exchanges of ideas, interchange of personnel and the world-wide sale of equipment by firms famous in many countries have led to an almost standardized body of knowledge throughout the world. Here and there other, older forms of treatment, ayurvedic medicine in India, the medicine man in Africa and among American Indians, acupuncture in China, have persisted and indeed have not been officially discouraged, on the principle that it is better to have some kind of recognized authority in matters of health than to have none at all. Modern cults have also developed: homeopathy is partly absorbed in the NHS in Britain; osteopathy has had official support in some parts of the US, and condemnation in others; and chiropraxis has practitioners in many places. Lesser cults, particularly those concerned with diet, also exist; and in all countries there is some folklore medicine, especially in rural areas.

None of these (except perhaps homeopathy) enters into any of the established health services or health insurance systems of the Western world or into the health care systems of the European communist countries. So when we talk of health care and medical treatment it is to the world-wide system as practised by medical men and women trained in medical schools and modern hospitals that we refer. That it is today scientifically based and that it is capable of further advances by research methods is generally accepted and nowhere is there any significant move away from it. In Britain modern care is the result of steady and continuous development of this system, and it is noteworthy that since 1858 the training of doctors, their fitness to practise, their continuing conformity to the rules, have been controlled by a statutory body, the General Medical Council. The GMC keeps a register of all men and women who have fulfilled the necessary curriculum of training and examinations and only those whose names appear on that register can in law act as medical practitioners.

So our system of medical care is part of the main stream of

medical knowledge: it is in the delivery of medical care that the UK system differs from others. But what has to be added to make it a complete system of health care? First, all the techniques and methods for the prevention of disease. Much has already been done but neither in their training nor by the way in which their work has been organized have the great bulk of doctors been vitally concerned with prevention of ill health. So far as we have tackled the problem it has been mainly through the work of the Public Health Service, and by its very nature that has been principally concerned with those infectious diseases in which immunization methods were applicable and in the care of mother and child. Prevention of other diseases must be an important part of any developing health service.

Part of prevention must be through the education of the public in matters of health and this is another formidable problem not well tackled in any western country. In the Soviet Union, on the other hand, there is actually a Ministry for Health Education, and great efforts are made to tell the people about health and what they must do to preserve and improve it. In this country, and most others, the doctors have not been trained in health education and any training they have received has been largely incidental. The methods of payment most common, fee-for-service, capitation and so on, are not conducive to disease prevention since they are all based on the treatment of ascertained disease. The family doctor, who should be the leader in this matter, has in the past been largely cut off from the health prevention team and it is only now as health centres increase in numbers that the health team is becoming established and made conscious of this problem. Society has, however, to play its part by insisting that those things known to be harmful are publicly pronounced upon and publicly condemned. But half-hearted efforts will not get rid of the deleterious elements in our environment, as can be seen in the case of cigarette smoking.

Public education will need to be intensive for the public tends to look for easy ways and does not like to be personally inconvenienced. Flaws in the environment, impure water or food, oil on our beaches, poisonous wastes in our streams will all be condemned by the whole population who will then expect experts to deal with them. But the things that will prevent disease in the individual, like the abolition of cigarette smoking, will need to be fought for very hard and will need the unanimous support of the whole medical profession. Techniques of explanation and persuasion now largely used by some of the people who purvey harmful substances will need to be adopted by a health care system dedicated to prevention.

The people will, however, also need positive education in matters of health, and this is still relatively rudimentary in most countries. On the one hand doctors have never agreed to educating even their own patients, and many would be reluctant to attempt to educate citizens in general. Nor is there a body of knowledge in simple form which can easily be used in all countries, and insufficient study has been made both as to what people must be told and on what subjects people want to be educated. The success of manufacturers of patent medicines, obtained by education through advertising, shows that the public can be persuaded, but new methods in public relations will be needed to achieve results.

One concept which has never been put to the people is that they have not only a right to health care but a duty to seek it. Beveridge touched on this in his Report. He was discussing the relationship between the payment of high benefits for disability and the need for the active co-operation of the patient to overcome that disability. 'It is a logical corollary,' he wrote, 'to the receipt of high benefits in disability that the individual should recognize the duty to be well and to co-operate in all steps which may lead to the diagnosis of disease in early stages when it can be prevented.' (He should, of course, have said 'treated effectively', since he is speaking of diagnosable disease.) Beveridge would not have gone as far as Samuel Butler in *Erewhon* where it was considered criminal to be ill, and he did not carry the argument as far as in Norway where it is said that 'the citizen has a legal and moral right to seek immediate medical aid for any ailment'. Certainly any discussion of the meaning of health must embody the idea of the sick having a duty to seek efficient medical aid in order to regain health as quickly and completely as possible. If we are ever to attain what was fashionably called, in the 1940s, 'positive health', the citizen must have a positive duty to seek aid and therefore a right to aid of the highest standard.

When we have educated the public and have prevented all the disease we can, will the effort and the money spent produce new expansions of life? On the purely material side will we spend less on medical care? Certainly in so far as education in health leads people to do all the things they can there will be less disease. The effects of a complete ban on smoking, of finding new ways to prevent accidents, in the home, in the factory and on the highway, the saving of suffering by earlier diagnosis of chronic diseases and other factors would all reduce our present disease and death levels. On the other hand, as we have already noted, saving of lives leads to an increase in the expectation of life at all ages and more people may survive with chronic conditions needing continuous treatment. It is impossible to draw up even a forecast budget, but it seems almost certain that costs in a comprehensive service will increase for years to come and society cannot look for financial savings within decades, probably not until the century is almost ended. But the advantages to State and individual should by then be obvious to all and the extra cost should be met from increasing affluence. That affluence should be accompanied by increasing leisure: and one task will be to find ways of using that leisure as part of the health programme.

Man has many disabilities and is subject to attack by many outside agencies but he also creates many new hazards for himself, and in an atomic age he has on balance probably produced more threats to his very existence than he has removed. As he continues to improve his technical medical care and increases his understanding of health he also faces world-wide problems of overpopulation, of possible universal hunger, of pollution of his whole environment. By AD 2,000 he will have to solve the problem of leisure, the problem of how to look after an increasingly aged population, and to rid himself of the dangers he has himself created. All these are matters of health, and health, that state of well-being however defined, will continue to be one of man's preoccupations. What must now be discussed is how all those involved – the individual, the community, the doctor, the health worker and administrator – can be given a unified outlook and a united purpose: the improvement and maintenance of the health of all human beings.

But one other point must be recognized. In describing and discussing how far along the road to a system of delivery for health care the nations have advanced we are in fact speaking mainly of a system of medical care, that is of care given by doctors, physicians and their associated ancillary and auxiliary aids to those suffering from disease. Disease, as the word implies, may be physical or mental or, as we know today, both; and it ranges from mild chronic conditions with no killing potential to catastrophic illness and accident, often fatal without medical care and frequently fatal in spite of all that is done. As we have already noted there is not one unified administrative structure in the way that there is a single body of medical knowledge, yet over the past fifty years a thread has continuously linked the thinking on how efficient delivery of all kinds of care can best be achieved. As Anne R. Somers, one of America's best students of health care, has said (*Modern Hospital*, vol. 115, no. 3 (Sept. 1970), p. 87): 'Public responsibility for assuring *equal* access to health services is taken for granted in most of Europe, as completely as responsibility for education and public safety.' Most countries indeed were trying to fulfil what is now the United

Nations view of health as a human right before that body was formed, and have gone on developing along similar lines.

It must also be clear that since then countries have gone ahead with organized government sponsored or controlled schemes, but once these are established the people must be satisfied that high standards can be and are maintained in such a service. Speaking of Norway on this point Karl Evang declared that 'medical care has reached the highest level of quality where prepaid medical systems have been fully developed.' The same can be said about most countries, and Anne Somers concluded from her own studies that 'the excellent showing of both countries [Sweden and England] in terms of comparative mortality and morbidity rates while not conclusive as to the superiority of their systems, certainly precludes any effort to identify public financing with poor quality care'.

Chapter 3

The United Kingdom

The development of health care in Britain has a very long and a very important history, important in the sense that innovation, observation and research have always been features of it and from them international recognition of British medicine has developed over the centuries. It was not in medical science alone that Britain advanced but on a broad medical and social front which spread from the provision of hospital care for the 'deserving poor' to schemes for pure water and pure food and for the protection of the child against the harshness of the industrial revolution. From the beginning of the nineteenth century the voices of reformers spoke of the need for medical care yet the first scheme of National Health Insurance was not introduced until 1911. That an ultimate solution to the problem of providing medical care would be a political one was clear to many from the beginning of the present century and the argument as to the form it should take went on continuously until the beginning of the NHS in 1948; and it has gone on ever since, because all the political points that had been made had not been answered. The service itself has been praised by many who have studied it from outside: it has been praised by the people of Britain in the way in which they have learned to use it. It stands at the head of those European systems that attempt to be comprehensible and universal. Its strengths may be an example to others, but its weaknesses call for further development within.

From the first definite call for a State medical service in the *Minority Report on the Reform of the Poor Law* (1908) to its inauguration, there were forty years of active discussion, but, more important, of change and development. From 1890 to 1910 all over Europe there was a surge of development in ways of providing and, above all, of paying for medical attention. A great part of this was among groups of workers, in areas where community concepts included medical care, and through governmental action, especially in Germany, where Bismarck regularized the growing system of sick clubs and gave them a form which still persists. The year 1911 was in some ways most significant, with countries as different as Norway and Britain introducing a system of health insurance to cover a section of the working population. It produced the first battle of a struggle between the community and the medical profession which still goes on, a struggle which must be ended in any future development of the present service. It was essentially, and still is, a rearguard action attempting to prevent the community from going forward on lines that seem to threaten the financial position of the medical profession. The first phase of the struggle, against the Lloyd George scheme of 1911, ended only, but abruptly, when more money was offered than had appeared likely in the early phases. That 'trade union' type conflict has been repeated many times and the doctors have always failed to hold up the new proposals but have usually secured an economic advantage for themselves.

No feature of the medical life of 1910 persists today: and when one considers the development in the ancillary health fields the difference is almost unbelievable. The general practitioner worked single-handed, his stethoscope almost his only essential piece of equipment, and his range of skills covering medicine, midwifery and a good deal of surgery. The specialist as we know him today existed in teaching hospitals only and even there his assistants were nurses, and technical experts were almost unknown. X-rays were still elementary and laboratory work was only just being accepted as an essential part of clinical medicine. The poor of Britain got some kind of care from the poor-law system of hospitals attached to the workhouses; while the voluntary hospitals provided a combination of charity and private practice medicine. In these circumstances it is surprising to find that far-seeing doctors were planning a health service. Dr Benjamin Moore in *The Dawn of the Health Age* (1910) and others were describing health centres in quite modern terms before World War I. Once National Health Insurance had become established, and as a larger and larger number of people came to be covered by it, new developments came along at regular intervals: a Minister of Health in 1919, the municipalization of the poor-law hospitals in 1931 and the establishment of what was virtually a national hospital service in 1939 to meet the needs of World War II. When the Labour Party won the first election after that war it was against a background of intense discussion, but also of consensus on the need for a universally available service. The principles that were then laid down were embodied in the National Health Service Act in 1946 and those principles remain in spite of some small departures, solely on the question of charges.

It is interesting that the Beveridge Report already quoted had dealt firmly with the two great principles, universality and comprehensiveness, but had left open the third, and in many ways the one that needs most emphatic statement and firmest adherence—that there shall be no financial barriers to any service any citizen requires. Beveridge said that he assumed 'that a comprehensive national health service will ensure that for every citizen there is available whatever medical treatment he requires, in whatever form he requires it, domiciliary or institutional, general, specialist or consultant, and will ensure also the provision of dental, ophthalmic and surgical appliances, nursing and midwifery and rehabilitation after accidents'. He insisted that this must be part of the overall social service but must be organized by 'departments responsible for the health of the people and for positive and preventive as well as curative measures'; and must be provided 'without contribution conditions', although he left others to decide 'whether or not payment towards the cost' be collected in some way. At the moment when Beveridge was writing that report he could quote from a British Medical Association document words that fully satisfied the Labour Party that the doctors would support a new health service. The Draft Interim Report of the BMA Medical Planning Commission accepted the need 'to provide a system of medical service directed towards the achievement of positive health, of the prevention of disease, and the relief of sickness: and to render available to every individual all necessary medical services, both general and specialist, both domiciliary and institutional'.

That is what Great Britain has today. Why then the need for new plans and fresh consideration of what was in 1946 both idealistic and practical and which has been described by an American writer, Almont Lindsey (*Socialized Medicine*, 1962), as 'one of the great achievements of the twentieth century'? The answer is twofold. Firstly the original plan did not match the principles with an administrative structure that would enable the ideals to be completely achieved, and secondly no structure could possibly meet all the new demands of a growing and developing science like medicine or meet the wishes of a public which has in the twenty-five years of the service learned not only its good points but its weaknesses and deficiencies. As we have seen, our UK health services have been reviewed periodically and changed at regular intervals and our democratic system calls for such a review now.

In practical terms what Britain has today is a service fully available to everyone living in the country at any moment, a comprehensive service in both terms of content and distribution but one which still has gaps in its provisions. It is a service which for diagnostic and curative medicine is based on the general practitioner or family doctor, from and through whom all the services relating to diagnosis and treatment are obtained and by whom, increasingly, preventive measures are given. The mass of preventive medicine, however, hygiene, immunization, care of the school child and so on are in the hands of special public health officers. The general practitioner advises on and arranges hospital care for his own patients: and the hospitals, organized locally and regionally, give every form of physical and mental care and employ the specialists who man all the different departments. Dental service, the provision of medicaments, testing of eyes and dispensing of spectacles are also included in the benefits of the service. It is part of the social security system but its finance is quite separate, and as Beveridge advised the right to the service is in no way tied to the payment of contributions. The freedom of doctor and patient are preserved, the citizen's to choose his or her own doctor, the physician's to prescribe everything he considers essential to his patient's welfare. In its twenty-five years of life the service has been controlled for eleven by its founders, the Labour Party, and for fourteen by the Conservative Party which in 1946 voted against it; but no serious voice has been raised suggesting that the principles of the service are wrong. As the cost of medical care has grown in the UK as everywhere else the great bulk of the money to meet it has come from general taxation.

So the service rests on the general practitioner and on the citizen's free choice of the doctor he wants to attend to him. When we discuss Europe as a whole in a later chapter we will describe how most countries organize their services around a man who is primarily a diagnostician, often the community physican and equally often the family doctor, a specialist in other words in the treatment of people in their own environment. In most countries, as here, the general services include not only the doctor but also the dentist, the pharmacist and the optician and are organized separately from the hospital service. Great Britain has approximately 20,000 general practitioners who on average look after 2,460 patients who have chosen them. Ninety-eight per cent of citizens have made the positive choice of a doctor which in some senses is equivalent to the exercising of their duty to seek treatment, which we discussed earlier.

We may look at the NHS in three ways. First, what does it mean in terms of money spent and in terms of what the nation gets. Other countries spend more but if their service is fragmented as in USA they do not get the value that comes from planning, coordination and spreading the risks on the whole nation. Table 3.1 shows the position in 1969 – a year which so far as possible will be used

Table 3.1 Health Service Resources (England and Wales, 1969)

Persons registered with a general practitioner	47,165,895
All general practitioners	20,208
Average doctor's list	2,495
Prescriptions during a year	245,539,000
Average cost per prescription	147.7*d.*
Sight tests per year	6,357,000
Eyeglasses dispensed	4,838,000
Dentists	10,659
Treatment courses by dentists	18,011,296
Dentures supplied	1,668,000

for statistics throughout this book – but gives only the figures and not the life-blood of a service. These show what the nation spends £2,000 millions a year on but that does not reflect the great services individuals have had. The finance comes from the following sources; approximately 5 per cent from charges, private bed fees and so on, 10 per cent from the weekly contributions made for social security as a whole and the rest, 85 per cent, from general taxation. The pattern of how it is spent remains fairly constant over the years as shown in Table 3.2 for 1969–70, with the hospital services taking

Table 3.2 Costs Met from All Sources of Finance (Great Britain, 1969–70)

	£ millions	*Per cent*
All services	1,952	100
Central government services	1,685	86.3
Central administration	11	0.5
Hospitals: Current	1,013	51.9
Capital	129	6.6
Executive councils		
Administration	13	0.7
General medical	143	7.3
Pharmaceutical	196	10.0
General dental	89	4.6
General ophthalmic	27	1.4
Welfare funds	40	2.1
Other	24	1.2
Local authority services		
Health	169	8.7
Welfare	98	5.0

the greatest proportion. In terms of resources and personnel the hospital service is a very large undertaking (Table 3.3). In all countries hospitals absorb most of the money spent on medical care and it is interesting to speculate, as we do later, on how much more value might be got from increasing the general medical

Table 3.3 Some Hospital Statistics (UK, 1970)

Number of beds available and staffed	513,000
In-patients discharged or died	6,028,000
New out-patients	9,279,000
Out-patients and casualty attendances	38,095,000
Consultants (as whole-time)	9,347
Other hospital medical and dental staff	17,946
Nurses (whole-time or part-time)	313,847
Domiciliary visits by specialists	318,000
Blood transfusion donations (bottles)	1,713,000

services which at present take a surprisingly low proportion of the total. The general medical services take only 7.8 per cent of the total and with dental and ophthalmic only a combined proportion of 13.9 per cent. It is somewhat unexpected to find that more is spent on drugs ordered by GPs than they themselves earn—10.1 per cent of the total.

From another angle it can be said that the nation gets its comprehensive service for less than £40 per annum per head of the population, an amount that compares very well with other countries. Of course any comparison of what is spent must also consider the services available and Table 3.4 indicates that Britain has very much

Table 3.4 Resources per 10,000 of population (1965 or nearest)

Country	*Doctors*	*Hospital beds*	*Dentists*	*Nurses and midwives*	*Pharmacists*
Belgium	12.5	82.0	—	—	—
Canada	11.7	110.0	3.0	77.4	4.1
Denmark	12.3	91.0	5.2	39.6	3.2
France	11.6	133.9	3.8	25.5	4.4
Germany (FRG)	14.5	107.0	5.3	27.1	3.0
Holland	11.2	75.7	2.3	12.0	1.3
Japan	10.9	—	3.5	26.5	7.0
Norway	12.0	106.2	7.2	32.0	3.4
Sweden	11.0	159.1	7.9	92.9	1.0
UK	11.5	105.5	2.7	26.0	3.1
USA	14.8	90.0	4.8	46.4	6.1
USSR	24.0	96.0	—	35.0	—

a middle place in regard to the biggest items. On the number of doctors per 10,000 of the population the UK is certainly not overstaffed but is below both the USA and the USSR. In terms of hospital beds Britain appears to have a good average figure but there is debate everywhere as to how many beds are needed for an efficient service. One thing the NHS has demonstrated is that hospital beds can be used efficiently and economically if empty beds and beds used by a patient longer than is necessary are eliminated. Since the NHS started the number of patients who receive in-patient treatment has gone from 3,750,000 to 5,970,000, although in the same period treatment in many fields, intensive care, new surgery and so on has become more complicated and more expensive.

There is no hard statistical way in which service benefit can be clearly identified and anyone studying this subject has to make up his mind how services compare on a great many factors and after viewing many institutions. What can be said is that in no feature do the UK services lag seriously behind any other country and on an overall average the nation gets a fairly comprehensive service, a fairly evenly distributed service and an above average level of medical skill.

The service must also be looked at from the patient's point of view. If we leave out of this action those preventive services and educational proposals which are of a community nature and remember that the average citizen hopes not to need medical care at all, what does the patient get? Above all, in Britain, from the moment he selects his general practitioner and as long as he remains a potential patient of the same doctor, he can get continuous personal attention of a general nature and the service of a physician who can arrange for any other kind of medical care that proves necessary. Much emphasis must be given to the concept of 'continuing care', for it is in direct contrast to the episodic care which a private fee-for-service system gives, as in the US. This is discussed further in Chapter 5 but it is the best part of the British service and of other European systems. It is also much more efficient and much more economic. If there is no 'physician of first resort' the patient has to attempt his own diagnosis and go direct to a specialist who is under pressure to take every case into hospital because most insurance covers hospital care but not continuing care by a generalist. One of the criticisms made about the British GP is that he does not spend so much time on his cases, does not do nearly so many laboratory tests (expensive) or X-rays (which can be dangerous if repeated). But Americans are astonished that British doctors do so many house visits and very envious of the unrequested calls elderly patients often get from their doctor. Of course if he sees his patients continuously he knows them, their history, their ailments, and does not need the elaborate and costly tests on which a doctor who sees people only for an episodic illness depends.

Since 1911 the people of Britain have known this kind of continuing service and while they may sometimes grumble and occasionally are fully justified in serious complaint, they know they now have a good service. What is more they have seen it grow and develop, they have heard doctors and politicians argue over it and its shortcomings and they find that the practitioner who does domiciliary visits, who knows the family and the environment, can be a very good friend as well as a good doctor. It must be noted that Britain has a more stable society than some other countries and so a high proportion of citizens do keep to the same doctor for many years, and mutual trust and understanding play a large part in the practice of National Health medicine.

It was, however, fully recognized in the debates on setting up the service not only that the general practitioner could not go on working single-handed, but that he had to be brought into the enlarged modern medical team. First he needed to be brought into some kind of organized group of GPs so that they could be of mutual assistance, could organize their work and could support one another during holidays and time off generally. Then these groups would have to work with and also guide all the other community health workers, nurses, midwives, health visitors and so on: and it was long ago seen that to do this doctors must be moved out of their individual 'surgeries' or offices, as some call them, and brought together in a health centre, the focal point, it was hoped, for all this work. The idea of health centres was first put forward as long ago as 1913 and from that date it gained increasing support. It was one of the tragedies of the NHS that national financial problems and political opposition made the provision of health centres very slow. The building of health centres is now more rapid but it is still a slow process. In Scotland, where they are built by the central government there were only 34 at the end of 1971 and it was estimated that early in the 1980s there would be 200. In England and Wales the buildings are put up by county councils; at the end of 1971 there were nearly 400 in use and it was projected that by 1980 there might be some 1,300. Unfortunately only a small proportion of those already in operation are built and staffed according to the original concept, so essential to the future development of health as distinct from medical care, with dental departments, pharmacy and all the necessary ancillary staff.

What the patient will get from a health centre in which there is real integration of a staff capable of giving a comprehensive service will obviously be very different from the service given by an individual doctor, and as the integration proceeds and as a sense of social responsibility pervades the whole team medical care will be greatly improved and health care will become a reality.

The third way in which what the citizen gets can be examined is from the point of view of administration. A health service should be under one administrative system, for neither disease nor the sick person is divisible. It has been possible, but far from ideal, to run the NHS in three parts with three quite separate organizations but this is really indefensible in a national, universally available service. It is generally accepted that the service needs a strong central body, the Department of Health, to indicate and control the national strategy for health; a regional body to do the broad planning; and local bodies to carry on the day-to-day work. There is no agreement as to how these bodies should be constituted but a plan of this kind is generally envisaged. It is what we have had since 1948 for the hospitals, regional hospital boards and local hospital management committees (in Scotland the structure and names are a little different). The service has been sharply split into this hospital structure and two other administration machines, that is executive councils, one for each county area, and the county and county borough councils in their capacity as local health authorities. The executive councils are responsible for all the 'general' medical services, the local authorities for the prevention of disease, the care of the child, domiciliary midwifery, the provision of health centres, ambulances and other community services. An indication of how NHS money is divided between these three sections is given in Table 3.2; Table 3.5 shows how the staff, almost one million, is divided between the three sections.

This division was contrary to the original intention of those who advocated the NHS and was a compromise reached at the time because the role, and even the geographic boundaries, of local government needed reform, because the doctors objected strongly to control by existing local authorities, and also because GPs had grown accustomed to their service being organized separately under the old National Health Insurance system. The executive councils were somewhat unique in our democratic society for the membership was fixed at an equal number of producers of general medical care, doctors, dentists, pharmacists and opticians, and of consumers of care, the general public. They were mainly devised from the same local authorities which controlled the preventive domiciliary and hygiene services. It is to be regretted that before such a major reform was undertaken there was no good and complete study of how these three bodies had functioned and whether one functioned better than another; and above all no study of which type of members worked best, the directly elected or the local authority, the indirectly elected on the executive councils or the appointed on regional boards and hospital management committees.

Table 3.5 Manpower in the NHS (1970, UK)

Hospital service		
Doctors and dentists (as whole-time)	27,301	
Nurses	313,847	
Midwives	19,601	
Professional and technical (as whole-time)	39,905	
Ancillary	260,249	
Administrative and clerical	50,451	
Other	12,035	
		723,389
Executive council services		
Doctors	24,458	
Dentists	11,936	
Ophthalmic medical practitioners	981	
Opticians	6,729	
Other	8,914	
		53,018
Local authority (health and welfare)[1]		
Doctors and dentists	1,488	
Nurses	25,908	
Home helps	37,720	
Social workers	7,077	
Ambulance	16,843	
Other	76,289	
	941,723	165,325

[1] The figures for local authorities are for England and Wales only and as whole-time equivalents.

This division in the system of administration has, over a period of twenty-five years, had the effect of preventing team work from developing as it should; it has not hastened the increase of services on a community basis or permitted experiments to see how much that is now done expensively in hospital could be better and more economically done in the community. In such a situation what should be done officially has to be tried out in differing ways in different places: and in some areas the domiciliary based services and the doctors in the hospitals have drawn closer than the administrative split would seem to make possible.

One important aspect of this increasing co-operation is the domiciliary consultation service under which in 1969 there were 318,000 cases in which the consultant visited a patient at home at the request of the GP. When this resulted in a decision that the patient could stay at home the saving on the hospital service was considerable; when the decision was that the patient should be taken to hospital at once, the citizen was getting a level of medical care unexcelled in any country. This co-operation between the family doctor and the hospital specialist must be increased and will be made very much easier and more effective when the services are managed by one body instead of two, and should be a greatly enhanced feature of medical care once all doctors become clearly what they now are in effect, salaried officers of one service.

Medically, socially and personally the vital aspect of the NHS is that in it medicine has been taken out of the market-place, has no financial barriers and enhances the freedom of doctor and patient alike to improve the standard of health in the country. The fees that have been introduced in dentistry, pharmacy, optics and so on are totally irrelevant to the total cost, some £50 million in all. They are merely a device for collecting a little money by a route other than general taxation, as is shown in Table 3.6. What is

Table 3.6 Sources of NHS Finance (1969–70, UK)

	£ millions	*Per cent*
All services	1,952	100.0
Central government	1,685	86.3
Consolidated funds	1,447	74.1
NHS contributions	175	9.0
Charges to recipients	59	3.0
Miscellaneous	4	0.2
Local authority		
Rates and consolidated fund grants	233	11.9
Charges to recipients	34	1.8

important is that the ordinary citizens, all of them, have a guaranteed system for the delivery of health care which is their right and for which the Government of the day is bound by law to make the necessary arrangements. There is one portal of entry to medical care, the general practitioner. On the one hand he has contracted to give all medical aid 'within his own competence' to those he has accepted as patients on his list. On the other he exercises on behalf of these patients their right to every form of hospital and specialist care, physical and mental. The people of Britain accept the NHS as part of their way of life but reserve their right to criticize and complain where it seems to fall below its own standards.

The Conservative Government also accepts that the NHS is essential to the well-being of the people of Britain. Earlier, in opposition, the Conservative Party voted against the principles of the NHS, but since it has been in power no such opposition has been voiced. The Secretary of State for Social Services, Sir Keith Joseph, has repeatedly confirmed his view that while modifications in how money for the NHS may be collected it has to be supported to the full. Speaking to a BMA meeting on 8 February 1972 he announced the provisional budget for five years, about £13,000 millions, and said, 'We have a potentially superb Health Service'. He claimed that the 'standards of specialist, general practice and community medicine are probably higher than in any other country in the world', and he went on to commit the Conservative Government to reorganize the service, for which we have found neither "the ideal balance between local initiative and central financial control, nor the ideal linkage between the interdependent worlds of local government and health services". That the system is nationally accepted and unlikely to change in basic principles was indicated by his going on to say that we have not yet 'evolved in all cases a sufficiently dynamic and yet sensitive system of responding to the infinite range of needs of patients and their relatives'. Sir Keith Joseph then described weaknesses which he wanted to remove and new demands which must be met to satisfy 'a population that is expanding and eager to benefit from rising medical standards'.

The fact that the people should be eager to use the service indicates how much it has already done. One may define it more sharply by another comparison with the USA. There the people have four main health fears: fear that they will not get medical aid when they need it; fear that having found medical aid they will not get all that is necessary because it is not provided or they cannot pay for it; fear that they will get too much, a fear based on the thought that when medicine is paid for by market-place methods doctors will be tempted to do unnecessary things to earn bigger fees; and the fear that no matter what insurance or other provision one has made, a serious illness will cost far more than the average person can afford. Apart from ordinary humanitarian principles, when one considers how much of ill health is psychosomatic, this freedom from fear is of enormous medical benefit to the sick.

Chapter 4

The Soviet Union

In any blueprint for health care account must be taken of the system developed in the past fifty years in the USSR. The greatest medical historian, Henry E. Sigerist, wrote in *Socialized Medicine in the Soviet Union* (1937), 'no one can deny that Soviet Medicine in the short period of twenty years and under most trying circumstances, has stood the test and has created powerful measures for the protection of the people's health'. Over twenty years later John Fry in *Medicine in Three Societies* (1969) wrote 'The USSR has developed an impressive system of medical care that is available and accessible to all. It has created tremendous resources of medical personnel, trained and in training, but there are problems relating to the fundamental structure'. As he goes on to say, the Soviet Union, immediately after the revolution, made health care one of its most urgent priorities but had to start from almost nothing; and so the service tended then, and the tendency persists, to follow a rigid pattern not well adapted to accepting new ideas and methods. Dr Fry's main criticism, and indeed that of most western observers, is on the question of the 'physician of primary contact', and whether he must be, as in British thinking, a well-trained specialist in primary care, which is how many GPs think of themselves. The USSR, without accepting the American idea of the patient's selecting and going to a specialist direct, has not kept to the concept of a general practitioner but has divided the duties of a primary care physician among a number of physicians and other health workers. Today the USSR has the highest number of physicians per unit of population of all countries, 70 per cent are women, and all work shorter hours than in capitalist countries. The divisions mentioned among the physicians of primary contact is somewhat like that in the USA, and is a division by age and sex and sometimes by type of therapy. While there is much talk in the USSR about the family as the essential unit of society, there are no family physicians. The care of the child is undertaken by doctors specialising in child health, and while this has given good results in that field it has meant a departure from the European single portal of entry to the health care system.

In looking at the USSR health services both Sigerist and Fry make the point that one must accept that 'medical care is planned and developed on socialist and economic philosophies . . . it is a part of the whole national socio-political programme'. In effect medical care is free to all when needed, with the same sort of exceptions as in the UK—payments for drugs and certain appliances. Medical care is available to all the 230 million citizens of the USSR and great efforts have been made to distribute care over even the most rural areas. The physicians who join this care are well trained and are working to that same common body of scientific knowledge as the rest of the northern hemisphere. Essentially doctors are trained as specialists, so that the primary care physician is a specialist in that field and has selected that field quite early in his training. Every doctor is trained in prevention and indeed the greatest emphasis in health propaganda is on prevention: yet curative and preventive medicine are seen as one and every effort is made to keep all doctors aware of this principle. When one recalls the great epidemics from which Russia once suffered one can accept that to reach health statistics comparable with other parts of the advanced world, as she has done, great preventive campaigns have had to be carried through. Without question, one feature in achieving good health records has been health education, in which all doctors take part, and the participation of the people in all health matters.

The centre of health care in the USSR is the polyclinic, a term covering a wide range of sizes from the small neighbourhood unit with usually a primary care doctor for adults and a paediatrician for the children, plus possibly a factory doctor and of course ancillary staff. Such a unit serves a population of around 4,000 and is geographical, that is there is no free choice for the people in the neighbourhood, but the USSR claims that they are true family physicians because they do frequent visits to the home. In a rural area there may be no fully qualified doctor but a staff of nurses and a midwife headed by a Feldsher. The Feldsher has clearly defined duties in preventive and diagnostic work and is in close touch with the doctors at the nearest fully staffed clinic or a district hospital. Ambulatory patients obtain their specialist care at the larger polyclinics, which vary in size but usually have at least surgeons, psychiatrists and specialists in ear, nose and throat, eyes, or other fields. In many urban areas the neighbourhood doctors work in the same polyclinic building as the specialists, so that co-operation is close. These specialists do not, however, have hospital duties.

Because of the existence of the polyclinics hospitals do not require out-patient departments but deal solely with in-patients. Again, one or more polyclinics may be built within or on the edge of the grounds of a hospital but the staffs are quite separate. Those accustomed to specialists who see patients in out-patient departments (or on a domiciliary visit), treat them in hospital and see them again in a series of follow-up attendances find a weakness in the Soviet separation of specialists into these two groups. In some fields it may not be vital but it is difficult to visualise a surgeon who operates but does not see his patients before or after surgery except in the hospital bed.

Hospitals throughout any of the Soviets are closely linked and have defined duties. There are small, mainly rural hospitals which even if they have only ten beds or so will be linked with a feldsher post. The chief hospitals serve a district but are equipped and staffed to deal with all except the most highly specialised treatments, heart, lung and brain surgery, for instance. These are dealt with at regional hospitals and institutes, the number depending on the size and population of the republic (the USSR, it should be recalled, is a federation of independent republics). In every district hospital there is a chief physician whose task is to co-ordinate all these curative services. He is also responsible for the programmes for health education, for the preventive services and for rehabilitation; and he has to organise that unique feature of Soviet medicine, the occupational and industrial services which have their working facilities inside those factories large enough to justify the staff, or in some areas at and through the polyclinics. Much care is given to workers without their having to leave their place of work and both day and night hospitals are provided in many places. In the five years from 1965 to 1970 the number of industrial health complexes was increased by 20 per cent and more are promised.

Within the Soviet system there is a chain of responsibility from the Minister of Health of the USSR through the Ministry of each republic to the regions, districts and neighbourhoods, mainly through the Chief Physicians at each stage. But most of the administration is at regional level where the chief medical officer of the region has a people's elected Executive Council. In each area there is also an appointed director of each speciality and he is responsible for seeing that the service not only runs smoothly but reaches the people. It should be noted that all health workers in the USSR join the one Medical Workers Union (over 5 million members) and that officers and committees of the union are consulted at every level. Committees at any level therefore include representatives of both the consumers and producers of health care.

The USSR system at one time had to be valued in relation to the past history of Russia and above all to the terrible conditions under civil war and revolution. Deaths from typhus were numbered in millions and cases of typhoid, cholera and smallpox ran into hundreds of thousands; syphilis, tuberculosis and deprivation accounted for millions of deaths. Recovery was slow but suffered another great setback when some 20 millions lost their lives in World War II. It is a measure of what has been done in twenty-five years that Dr Fry in the book already quoted can without hesitation put the USSR, USA and UK into one comparative table from which Table 4.1 borrows some figures. From these and many others and

Table 4.1 Maternity Statistics Compared

	Birth rate per 1,000	*Maternal mortality per 100,000 births*	*Infant mortality per 1,000 births*	*Deliveries in hospital per 100 births*	*Average stay in hospital (days)*
USSR	18.4	32	28	100	8–9
USA	19.4	31	25	100	3–4
UK	18.4	25	20	75	7–8

from personal observation one can safely say that the USSR citizen is getting a high level of modern health care. In the five-year plan 1971–5 great spending on new hospitals and polyclinics is provided for by the earmarking of thousands of millions of roubles. Dr Boris Petrovsky, the Minister of Health, has asked for over 500,000 more hospital beds and 500 polyclinics.

But what special points should we note for our own planning consideration? Undoubtedly the great spending on child care has produced the most spectacular results. As Dr Petrovsky says in *Public Health in the USSR* (1970): 'The primary aim of maternity and child care is the prevention of disease'. The pregnant woman is granted 112 days of maternity leave with full pay: post-natal care is provided by more than 20,000 welfare centres and polyclinics. The newborn child comes at once under the care of paediatricians and district nurses and remains under their care until he is 15. The childhood epidemic diseases are now reduced to the low figures comparable with other countries. Petrovsky claims that all the care given means 'the children are taller, sturdier and the mortality rate among children of all age groups is decreasing'. There is still a need for special sanatoria for children suffering from forms of rheumatic disease, tuberculosis and other disabilities and these are provided in many parts of the country.

In other ways the Soviet system shows high spots in emergency care and the treatment of injuries. There is an excellent ambulance service and in many of the sparsely populated areas planes, helicopters and motorised sleighs are used. But the Russians have more than an ambulance service. It is a fully comprehensive emergency service through which every kind of emergency care is given, for injuries, burns, poisoning, sunstroke, but also for heart attacks and other emergencies. The emergency service handles about 30 million calls each year. The doctors and nurses who work in this service have been more and more highly trained and are specialists in emergency work. For a major disaster this service could rush teams of doctors and nurses to the spot in vehicles equipped to deal with loss of blood, heart failure or any kind of injury: and cases, especially in the great cities, are taken direct to the appropriate special hospital. As already mentioned special polyclinics serve large factories, that is those with over 800 workers (or fewer if there are special hazards, for example chemical). Rehabilitation of workers through spa treatment is a prominent feature not found anywhere else.

The boast of the USSR is that it has carried into effect its own Constitution which says that all citizens have a 'right to maintenance in old age and to . . . free medical service and the provision of a wide network of health resorts for the use of working people'. In building up the service the doctors have played a dominant role but it must be emphasised they have done so in accordance with the socialist principles of the Constitution, under which there should be complete identity of purpose. There is now one overall national plan in which 'all the public health bodies are headed by doctors'. The democratic nature of the system however, 'enables wide sections of the public to take an active part in the work of public health bodies. Each polyclinic, hospital or any other medical institution has a public council', elected by the people. It is of deep interest that the Soviet Union expects its doctors to understand their social responsibility which is, of course, easier in the absence of private practice. And the head of the system, the Minister of Health, is always a working doctor. The present Minister, Dr Petrovsky, still works as a surgeon. He himself believes that 'health protection and promotion are the responsibility and concern of both the authorities and the people'.

Chapter 5

The United States of America

In population the USA is the same size as the USSR. In health care it is so different that at first sight it would seem wrong to make the assertion of the last chapter, that these countries and others in the northern hemisphere are working to the same common body of medical knowledge. The Minister of Health of the USSR claims that the highest standard of that medical knowledge is 'available and accessible to every citizen of the USSR'. The President of the US declares that there is a crisis in health care in his country and calls for drastic changes. A few years ago Dr Walter J. Lear, in *Medical Care and Family Security* (1962), could say: 'In America today we know more than ever before how to prevent, diagnose and treat disease . . . but the gap between what *can* be done and what *is* done continually widens. . . . We *know* more than we *do*. We suffer from the tragedy of unused medical knowledge'.

Yet America spends more money on health than any other nation, 7.1 per cent of its Gross National Product in 1970, compared with 6.0 per cent in the USSR, 5.5 per cent in Sweden and 5.1 per cent in the UK. The cost of medical care in America has increased far more rapidly than the general inflation would justify reaching 7.4 per cent of the GNP in 1971: but as there is no system which guarantees care to all citizens the gaps and difficulties multiply and every study of health care in America reveals just how many people fail to get care, do not get the right care or the right amount of care or may find themselves facing enormous bills for the care they have received. There was great complacency among all but the poorest of Americans until Presidents, the Press and the mass media generally began to repeat over and over again what a poor showing the US makes in world health statistics. When a TV network showed a programme called *Don't get sick in America* and the press followed with detailed analysis of the situation, public opinion began to swing towards some kind of national plan for health care.

We have seen how the USSR service is said to fit socialist principles and how doctors are supposed to accept social responsibility.

In the USA doctors are supposed to fit into the American way of life, to engage in free enterprise, enabling their patients to make a choice within a host of competing individuals and institutions. When this matter is discussed in medical meetings many will agree that the ideal system for medicine might be one in which all fees had been abolished and a truly Hippocratic system introduced, but this is dismissed as utopian and 'contrary to our way of doing things'. It is in fact claimed by many doctors that medicine must continue on market-place principles and the doctor be the sole arbiter as to what is a fair fee for his own particular skill. Nevertheless as insurance has grown and broadened doctors have been increasingly prepared to accept payment from third parties, insurance plans and companies and the state under a variety of schemes. Millions of Americans, however, now get free medical care of sorts because they are poor and therefore 'medically indigent' or because they are over a certain age. Senior citizens may be provided with a substantial part of the cost of hospital care, but the scheme includes deductibles and exclusions and so is far from complete. The elderly may also have paid insurance to meet doctors' fees. Mal-distribution of medical care, however, is such that none of the devices tried can ensure that any particular form of care, general or special, is in fact available and accessible in every area. Local wealth, local geography and innumerable social factors all interfere with the distribution of doctors and other health workers. America is also short of every kind of health worker. She has absorbed thousands of foreign doctors, mainly from poor, underdeveloped countries, yet is said to need another 50,000 physicians to approach a good distribution. As a result there is much discussion (and some actual schemes) of the need to train a new kind of substandard physician, primarily to assist qualified doctors but already, and certainly in the future, competing in the medical field.[1]

Maldistribution means concentrations of doctors and services in the areas where the highest income groups live and conversely that in the areas with the greatest density of people services will be poor. The American nation seems to have been astonished in recent years to discover how closely linked are poverty and ill health. The experience of the Office of Economic Opportunity (OEO) seems to have surprised many. Established and financed to deal with poverty and to attempt to give deprived families an equal opportunity, through education and training, to fit into modern American life,

[1] In any case no direct comparison can be made between this proposed para-medical working in private enterprise medicine and the Feldsher working in a national service.

from the outset OEO found it could not deal with poverty without first dealing with ill health, and today it has nearly seventy centres at which the poor of the neighbourhood receive their health care. This experience epitomises another aspect of health care in the US, the identification of a problem is followed by an *ad hoc* organisation to deal with it. The system of 'funding', which is the usual way of referring to payment by the Government, makes this technique the easiest, but not necessarily the most secure, method by which money can be obtained to meet a newly discovered need. There are, of course, obvious groups like Indians on reservations and Eskimoes for whom special services have to be provided, but there are now nearly 300 categories of US citizens who are eligible for all or some medical care paid for by governmental funds. President Nixon has declared that 'the nation faces a massive crisis in health care' and said that both administrative and legislative action would be needed 'within the next two or three years' if a breakdown of the medical care system was to be avoided. His own proposals would however simply continue the identification of categories of people who could get free or subsidized medical care, going on with what Senator Edward Kennedy called 'the same sort of patchwork approach we have been using for too long'. It was the categorization of citizens which led Senator Kennedy, speaking to the Senate on 25 January 1971, to demand 'a more coherent health care system in place of divided and categorical approaches that have been tried under Government or private sponsorship in the past', and which have met 'with uniform frustration and defeat'.

It is strange that an affluent society which beyond question boasts some of the most advanced technological medical facilities in the world should nevertheless suffer from 'frustration and defeat' in its attempts to provide a system for the delivery of health care. It is this 'patchwork approach' which makes any attempt to describe the US situation almost impossible, for the number and variety of services, the range in quality and in cost, the geographical and various other problems all have to be considered. After visiting innumerable institutions ranging from a 'free clinic' to a university medical centre or the Mayo Clinic one realizes that there are still bound to be experiments going on in health care that have been missed.

Experimentation is an outstanding feature of the US medical care scene but it is in itself another proof of the failure, over all, of orthodox 'fee-for-service' methods, no matter how sophisticated in economic terms or how well equipped they may be. The experiments range from the 'free clinic' set up by students at some 140 centres, to try to give a resemblance of medical care to the students themselves in the first instance, to the drug addicts in particular, but spreading into services for anyone who is deprived, right up to the large schemes of prepaid medical care. Of these the Kaiser (Permanente) schemes have 2 million members and expensive hospitals and clinics. Nowhere else in the world have the trade unions had to attempt so much in this field. It is at least fifty years since trade union leaders realized that their members were not getting health care and began to demand its provision. Many unions, notably the International Lady Garment Workers, the Teamsters, the United Automobile Workers, the United Mineworkers, and the Clerks (Distribution Workers) built and still run their own clinics and hospitals: but they cannot cover all their members since they do not live in a closed community. Unions therefore also negotiate with employers to get money paid into a special fund, often managed by a joint committee, to pay for necessary care for their members, care which they may buy on the open market or through contracts with existing medical facilities. Experience of these and other devices has convinced the trade union movement that its members and their dependants will get adequate guaranteed nation-wide medical cover only inside a universal system. Today the AFL-CIO is the leading force in demanding a universally available system, the spade-work for which was begun by the late Walter Reuther of the Auto Workers.

It is the unions' scheme translated into legal language which a large group of Democratic Senators and Congress members are backing, the struggle spearheaded by Senator Edward Kennedy and Congresswoman Martha Griffiths. Together they hope that the 93rd Congress will end the crisis of health care and bring health security to all Americans. It is this word security that all protagonists of universal health care use, for the one thing Americans have not had is security, and many of the social ills of the US, the violence, the drug problem, the high murder rate in cities, arise from a general sense of social insecurity. 'For millions of our citizens', Edward Kennedy has said, 'health care of any sort is simply not available at any price. For millions more the quality of care available is so poor that it may fairly be said that the citizen will be worse off because of his contact with the system'. There is scarcely an American who has not experienced this absence of care or has not had to pay very dearly for what can be found. This is not solely a question of money. The health crisis 'affects rich and poor, black and white, old and young, urban and rural alike': all of which is reflected in those statistics which now horrify Americans, that in infant mortality the US trails behind twelve other countries, in expectation of life behind seventeen countries and so on. Private practice, based almost entirely on specialization and high fees, has failed to affect these and other figures.

So people have turned to insurance which also fails: '. . . it fails to control costs. It fails to control quality. It provides only partial benefits, not comprehensive benefits, acute care not preventive care. It ignores the poor and the medically indigent'. Health insurance is big business and the private companies make great profits, but health insurance pays only one-quarter of the health care bill. The patient, even with insurance has to pay large sums from his pocket, and, frequently, to run into debt. The large mutual funds like Blue Cross find themselves covering the old and the chronic sick, but quite unable to control escalating costs of hospital care. Besides, nearly all insurance is for hospital costs, a fact which compels doctors and patient alike to use hospital beds in a wasteful, inefficient and expensive way. Neither out-patient nor domiciliary service is developed, nothing at all like our British 'open access' to laboratories and X-ray departments. Costs are not examined as they are in Britain because they are all passed on to the patient, the insurer or the Government. Strangest of all, as Kennedy has pointed out, 'Unnecessary surgery is encouraged; far more surgery takes place in the United States than in other nations with far better health records'. The stories an observer hears about surgery not justified on clinical grounds and the work the Tissue Committee does in every hospital to try to curb this are quite astonishing. The figures cover every kind of operation but are especially striking for female surgery, and for procedures like circumcision, appendectomy and tonsillectomy.

Everyone points out, of course, that America has spent very large sums on medical research and her scientists have won many Nobel Prizes: many hospitals are staffed and equipped for every advanced technique known, but neither of these is enough. A modern society is bound to develop internal insecurity if its people know that some highly expensive hospital can do everything the rich request or need while the majority of the people do not get even simple domiciliary care. America's greatest weakness is that she has turned to 'specialists' without any clear definition of their standing or any statement as to the ethical basis on which they should work, and has turned away from the general practitioner. It is only half true that the people have turned away. They have been partly persuaded and partly compelled by the medical profession which in its adherence to private practice has gone out for the higher fees which the specialist can claim. Highly specialized doctors need highly specialised hospitals and in them costs have steadily risen 'progressively pricing more and more medical care beyond the reach of more and more people'. Rising costs and specialization have not been a feature of America alone, but in most other countries new systems of health care were brought in to deal with the problem, health insurance among them. From time to time individual doctors and politicians tried to get America to deal with the problem, but 'the United States alone stood apart from these world-wide developments'. As we have already said, 'America preserved its faith in the private sector . . . we left basic planning and development of health care to professional leadership and to the play of the market-place'. Yet America could not entirely ignore those poor and needy whom the Statue of Liberty had beckoned, and so 'although government did become involved in the effort to upgrade health care, the effort was always limited, categorical and inadequate'.

We have noted that the British Medical Association sometimes opposed advances in health care but also proposed changes; and on the continent of Europe physicians were often in the vanguard of health insurance reforms. The history of the American Medical Association is quite different. For nearly fifty years it has repeatedly taken a stand against advances, and since World War II has not merely been obstructive but has actively worked against any suggestion of changes that were even remotely like a departure from the free enterprise system. It has spent very large amounts of money in active hostility to all moves towards governmental action in health, and has used in its propaganda stories and statements about the health care systems of other countries that have been far from accurate. So strong has been the AMA opposition that Senator Kennedy was moved to tell the Senate that 'the crisis today reflects the fact that professional leadership alone was not capable of meeting the national needs, and that the demands and needs of medical care do not lend themselves to satisfaction solely through the forces and the dynamics of the market-place'.

One result has been, as already noted, the virtual disappearance of the family physician. He has been replaced by what can only be called 'specialoids'. There are a number of these, each of whom may deal with a different member of a family. There are general practitioners in small towns and rural areas but they are a declining force. In urban areas the children may be looked after by a pediatrician, but the term does not indicate the training and experience of the consultant pediatrician in Britain or the children's doctor in the USSR. The rest of the family will call on the kind of doctor they think appropriate, depending on what their own diagnosis is. The obstetrician and gynecologist may appear an easy choice but individuals call on other kinds of surgeons, dermatologists, psychiatrists, ophthalmologists and so on. For those who know they cannot pay the fee they will be asked for, the physician of first contact must then be whoever is on duty at the nearest emergency room in a local hospital; but what kind of service they get and whether a fee will be asked will depend on many variables. There is great difficulty in places in staffing emergency rooms and many of the doctors are trainees and often foreigners. There is even in some places a purely commercial type of service in which for the right to charge fees to third parties, insurers, the Government and so on, a group of doctors take over the emergency room.

One feature of this type of medicine is that it is episodic and there is no continuity, as there is in a system of primary care physicians under contract to give a service to a group of patients. Episodic care tends to be much more expensive because every new doctor requires to have a whole host of laboratory tests done: and X-rays are much more frequent, and potentially dangerous, than in systems where the personal doctor has his records and memory of what has been done over the years. Even when the patient receives hospital care there may be no continuity, for he does not so much attend his community or district hospital as go where his episodic physician or surgeon happens to have the use of facilities. Naturally there are towns of such a size that much of the medical care is channelled through one hospital and a degree of continuity is reached, but this is far from being the invariable rule.

Hospitals are the main focus for medical care even when groups of specialists have combined to use one building, variously named, for all their offices. The hospitals of America cover a very wide range in size, from thousands of beds down to little local units in rural areas. Their origins stretch from the old poor law, now the county medical services, to every kind of voluntary and charitable institution, and to places run for profit. Ownership runs from the individual, the company of doctors, religious foundations, to teaching hospitals and great private clinics. In brief it can be said that of America's 1,600,000 beds over 600,000 are in mental hospitals, almost 100 per cent under public control. Of the other beds government agencies own 60 per cent but these are almost entirely for the chronic sick and the poor, and handle only about 30 per cent of the admissions. The basis of staffing is equally varied. Those hospitals owned by the Federal Government, by a state or a county may have salaried whole-time staffs. The voluntary hospital, whether it charges patients or not, will be staffed by those doctors who have sought and obtained permission to use the hospital beds. They may or may not give some free care to non-paying or emergency cases and their number is sometimes as great as the number of beds. The definition of specialist has, therefore, none of the connotations familiar in the UK and other countries where the recognition of the specialist depends on his appointment to a particular post and itemized duties. The American specialist holds a certificate from the appropriate specialist board but that does not carry with it a hospital post. There are some specialists, in the laboratory, for example, who are appointed and who may or may not confine themselves to hospital duties. But even these may be paid by a sliding scale according to the number of tests done.

The fact that the Government had to step in and through Medicare and Medicaid provide for the financing of care for the elderly and the poor respectively does not affect the hospital position for staffing, planning or control. Like other categories Medicare is more a system for paying for care than for planning it or guaranteeing it: the patient still makes his own decision as to which specialist is needed. Medicare pays a substantial proportion of the cost of hospital care. If the patient has paid co-insurance for the purpose or is medically indigent, then doctors' fees may be met in whole or in part.

The story of Medicare and Medicaid will illustrate the difficulties that arise with categorical and non-comprehensive schemes. One major problem has been that for Medicaid each state has to introduce its own scheme and inside five years all have had to be cut drastically. In general, as Selig Greenberg has said in *The Quality of Mercy* (1971), 'Medicare falls far short of need. The biggest gaps are those of out-of-hospital drugs and dental care, which are not covered at all. On the average *Medicare meets only about 45 per cent of the total* health care expenditure of the aged.' The Medicare program has also been cut, through increased deductibles and copayments as well as increased premiums for medical fee insurance. Both schemes, Greenberg goes on, have been 'a veritable bonanza for the medical profession by enabling doctors to charge high fees for elderly and low income patients whom formerly they had often treated at reduced fees or free of charge'. Yet in spite of this Medicaid 'remains poor house legislation'.

These schemes are national schemes initiated by the Federal Government but operated through each state's Department of Health and Public Welfare. The Federal health services are controlled by the Department of Health, Education and Welfare, which is under a Secretary who is a member of the Government. There is no Minister of Health but an Assistant Secretary whose deputy is the Surgeon-General, a full-time civil servant and always a doctor of wide experience. There is a chain of regional offices which in future may play a part in planning and budget control of any new service. Hospital development has been influenced since 1948 by the Hill-Burton Act, a Federal program which contributes matching funds for building and hospital renovation in areas in which facilities are below average standards.

The United States has some 7,000 hospitals but it is estimated that $6 thousand million are needed for new hospitals and $10.5 thousand million for modernizing older hospitals. The extent to which these estimates are too high is difficult to assess because of two opposing factors: the over-use of hospital beds engendered by the insurance schemes which concentrate on bed costs; and the opposite factor that, just because of the cost – in 1972 as high as $120 a day for a private room – the length of stay in American hospitals is shorter than in most other countries. This is not necessarily a sign of efficient bed use when it is dictated by financial issues which may even override clinical needs. Most studies, however, demonstrate that the over-use factor predominates. Thus the Report of Federal Employees Health Benefit Program for 1966 shows (Table 5.1) that

Table 5.1 Surgical Procedures per 1,000 Persons Covered by Different US Schemes (1966)

Prepaid group Practice programmes	31.1
Employee organization Plans	56.7
Blue Shield plan (physicians' fees)	72.4

there is a very large difference, and clearly not a clinical difference, between groups of similar citizens according to how they obtain hospital care—by prepaid mutual schemes, by employee plans or by Blue Shield plans which pay the doctor for what he does. A writer in the *New York Times* (9 August 1971) put it another way. In the US, 'there may be too much medical care, rather than too little. The US has twice as many surgeons per capita as England and Wales and these American doctors perform twice as many operations as their British counterparts'.

The same writer put the converse, that some get too little health care, as one of America's biggest problems: 'According to some estimates between 35 and 45 million Americans, mainly members of minority groups living in ghetto and rural settings . . . are not receiving adequate medical care'. Since unemployment shot above

6 million and now includes many people from the formerly high income groups in aeronautics, those figures are too low; and for those who get no service or get partial service paid for out of Federal, state and local funds, the figure is probably 70 million. Insurance is very much an income-controlled question. Thus while only 11 per cent of these with incomes between $7,000 and $9,999 have no hospital insurance, 64 per cent of those under 65 with incomes less than $3,000 have no cover. The writer in the *New York Times*, however, had in mind among the most deprived the Chicano and Indian populations whose bad health record and lack of service is reflected in a life expectancy of only forty-two years, and the migrant workers, at least one million, for whom no health provision was made until the United Agricultural Workers Union set up its own clinic at Delano, in California.

At the other end of the scale there is one large category for whom the Federal Government spends about $1,500 million each year to provide completely free health care, the Veterans, all who have ever served in the armed forces. The Veterans Administration owns some 170 hospitals, many large and modern, and at least 100 clinics and other facilities. All these are staffed, as are many hospitals belonging to the various armed forces, by full-time officers and the standard of many is very high indeed, not only in treatment, but also in research. In any plans for a future health service these and other facilities which are publicly owned will play an important part.

Many people see the greatest hope for US medical care in the growth of prepaid health insurance plans, and indeed, the Kennedy-Griffiths Bill would give them a prominent part in the working up of a new system for a comprehensive service. There are a variety of these schemes, the Group Health Co-operative of Puget Sound being the best of those in which consumer and producer truly co-operate: the Community Health Association sponsored by the United Automobile Workers in Detroit; the Kaiser scheme, started by an employer but now very much controlled by the doctors in it; and the Health Insurance Plan of New York, started in 1947 by the city administration and now serving 760,000 people. All of them give a comprehensive service on a prepaid basis. These services are not all complete and are in no way identical, but they are capable of expansion and certainly capable of fitting into a national health insurance plan such as is now proposed.

In speaking of the opposition of organized medicine, through the American Medical Association, to advances in health care delivery, it should have been noted that from the start it opposed the Kaiser and all other prepaid health care programmes. Today there are still sixteen States which prohibit any attempt to set up prepaid services similar to that operating at Puget Sound. The AMA condemned this way of health care as unethical and managed to bar doctors who joined such a scheme from hospitals and even from certification as specialists, no matter how high their qualifications were. Today no one outside a narrow group of medical entrepreneurs would suggest that practising medicine without charging fees is 'unethical'. The opposite view is increasingly held in America as elsewhere.

The question of making this type of prepaid service legal in all states is so important that the Kennedy-Griffiths Bill would give the President an overriding power to declare such bodies acceptable under the new scheme; and not only acceptable but ranking first for any money allocated to a region or state. In so far as Senator Kennedy wants any new service to be efficient and economic the lessons learned from the Group Health Co-operative are having a profound effect. Their prepaid insurance covers ambulatory care at hospitals (and home calls) and aims at keeping hospitalization as low as possible. A writer in *New Republic* on 18 December 1971 said that 'while the national per capita cost of health care was $226 in 1970, for GHC members it was only $143. The biggest savings were in hospital expenses which averaged $27 per GHC member compared to $112 nationally'. But the writer, Peter Barnes, rightly said that the Co-operative gives a far wider cover than any other plan, including such unusual benefits as birth control pills and dietary supplements and world-wide insurance cover. Some fees are charged, for example for full maternity care or abortions, with the idea of preventing 'in and out membership'. And this really comprehensive service is given by dedicated doctors who, on a salary basis, are very well paid.

This is a necessarily brief summary of the US position. It is complicated and often obscure; it is divisory and categorical. Dr John Fry found little true collaboration between public and private sectors. He wrote: 'It is not surprising, therefore, with this diversity of responsibility that there is little evidence of co-ordination and collaboration between the public health and local government services and the non-government medical services which provide private medical care'. With such diversity, with so much emphasis by the medical profession on fees and payments, with the absence of continuing care by a physician of primary contact, many American writers are saying as Selig Greenberg does, 'Many of our doctors may be the best in the world. But in health care we are still a backward country'. No one accustomed to the European and British systems could reach any other conclusion: but the moment is ripe for great changes in the USA and when the Americans catch up with a system for the universal provision of comprehensive care their technological skill should give them a service which other nations will have to strive to equal.

Chapter 6

European Health Care Today

Health care in Europe began to assume an insurance and mutual aid basis soon after 1880 and has continued to be financed and controlled in that form, extending and expanding at differing rates in the different countries and, inevitably, requiring and gaining increasing central government support. While the variations are still considerable it is quite realistic to speak of European health care collectively and to contrast it with the systems described in earlier chapters. There are slightly differing attitudes to the subject, differences in the extent to which the citizen and the State are thought to have rights and duties in the field of health, and differences also in the attitudes, past and present, of the medical profession. Differences occur in training of health personnel but it is safe to say that all doctors are working within that large body of common knowledge about which we have already commented. In writing of the US no mention was made of Canada, which in its latest plans may be said to fit into the European type of service. The former Prime Minister of Canada, Lester Pearson, made it quite clear that policy 'would be directed to ensuring that all Canadians can obtain health services of high quality according to their need and irrespective of their ability to pay'.

Before writing of individual countries it is possible to make some general observations. None of the countries in NATO, or the Atlantic Community as it is called in its non-military aspects, can be said to be satisfied with their health care systems as they stand at present. All are in a state of constant re-examination, and all have over the years been approaching the position of having covered over 90 per cent of their people by schemes which are sometimes anachronistic in the way they work because of their history. Germany has perhaps the most rigid system, Norway the most flexible, but all are concerned with ensuring that they have achieved the best possible arrangements. Financing is a major problem and has two aspects. All countries are faced by the quesion of how much, in relation to national wealth and to spending on other services, they should spend on health care; and by the second question, of how the money is to be collected. The nearer to a service for 100 per cent of the people any country comes, the more attractive a simple straightforward taxation system becomes. There is political pressure in most countries both to increase the amount spent and to finance more and more of the service by a direct taxation method; and at the other end of what is often a complicated chain of personal payments followed by re-claim from an insurer, there is the demand to get rid of both the trouble and the bureaucracy such a method produces.

The health provision of all European countries is part of a wide ranging social security and social benefits system. Only in Britain have service benefits been entirely divorced from money benefits. But NATO countries are finding that the right to health care should be entirely free of fee-for-service insurance arrangements and so on, while money benefits should be contractual. In all schemes, of course, provision has to be made for the poor, and since the poor are never healthy and so must be encouraged, indeed exhorted to seek medical aid, it is better to have a universal system and not to have to provide separately for the poor. In Portugal, for example, the health insurance scheme applies only to the middle income range: the rich can provide for themselves, the poor are provided for by charity, the Church and by a poor-law system.

All European countries are caught in arguments about the primary care physician and most agree that a doctor of primary contact, a general practitioner, in other words, is essential. In discussions as to how this work is to be organized it is clear the British concept of group practice within health centres is gaining ground. But in an arctic country like Norway the primary physician has often to be the prevention and hygiene officer and the administrator within his community. This and other needs raise the whole question of community medicine, of the relation of the physician to his community, and of the degree to which citizens and physicians have to co-operate to get the best service. Many want to see much closer co-operation and doubt whether health insurance gives the most suitable financial basis.

Health insurance in Europe began in Germany under Bismarck. It had its origin (and still retains the principle) in sick funds which had an element of social security in their work. Bismark did not invent the idea but regularized and organised a movement which was growing among the workers in their efforts to get some form of health care. All the other European countries followed Germany at intervals, usually, as in Britain, with partial schemes covering only a part of the population and then taking in more groups of workers, agricultural, for example, and often throwing the system open, on a voluntary basis, for even the higher income groups. Today Germany has sick fund insurance which is compulsory for all wage earners and salaried workers below a certain income level. Some funds take in groups above that level and there are private sick funds for richer citizens; and altogether at least 90 per cent of the people are in some kind of scheme. The sick funds are supervised by the Federal Republic of Germany but administration is in the hands of the provincial governments.

Because of this, spending is not uniform and most areas have to be subsidized from the centre. Control is very much in the hands of a hierarchy of medical officers of health who also deal with all the sanitary, hygiene and prevention services which are local council responsibilities. From the start the German system was based on the general practitioner and this is still the case. A doctor has to have had three years' experience and a special course of training; he then joins a local doctors' association which enters into contracts with the sick funds. The sick funds pay a lump sum to the association which divides it among the doctors, according to the amount of work each claims to have done. Although the money is collected from employers and employees on a scale graduated according to salaries, all dependants are also covered, and the patient is free to choose a GP or a specialist from the published list of eligible doctors. The sick funds pay for X-rays, laboratory tests and so on, but there is no organized service for these aids which may be obtained from university or other hospital units or from private diagnostic centres. The latter are often financed by the doctors who are also the customers.

The German system also covers hospital care but there is a limit of eighteen months' hospitalization and the sick funds employ doctors to check on long-stay cases. Hospitals are largely publicly owned but there are still a number which are privately owned. Private practice, as seen in the USA, is almost non-existent and most specialists are salaried officers, only the chief of a unit being free to do private work. The German system appears inflexible and its standards are exceedingly variable, but it falls into the insurance based type of service without all the problems of deductibles and payments by the rich found elsewhere. On the whole Germany has well-distributed services and since dental and eye care are included the service is fairly comprehensive.

SCANDINAVIA

The five countries of Scandinavia have established a Nordic Council with the idea of keeping their health care systems developing along similar lines, making it possible for the citizen of any of the five to get comparable care in the others, and for doctors to work in all of them. Finland lags behind the others, having come into the health insurance field later. Their chief medical officers meet at regular intervals and they have in operation a similar list of drugs. The attitude in all these countries is very much towards a positive health programme and the people seem to understand their services and the reasons for their existence. The medical profession has played a vital part in the development of the new ideas and new services. Today all the Scandinavian countries have services that cover practically the whole of their peoples and are imbued with ideals best enunciated by Norway's Director General, Dr Karl Evang. 'The main goal' he says, 'is to provide every sick and infirm person with all the help and support which medical science can give for his particular need, not to make him a passive individual who must be permanently supported by others, but to aid him in becoming an active and happy member of society.' The Norwegian people have accepted this positive attitude to health and all want to see their country's health record improved, 'although Norway ranks high among the nations of the world measured by the usual yardsticks of average life-span, infant morality and occurrence of communicable diseases'.

Norway, Denmark and Iceland adhere more closely to a general practitioner type of service than does Sweden, where the provision and planning of modern hospitals has led to some extent to the populace looking to the local hospital as the focal point for medical care. All these countries began forms of health insurance for working people as part of general social insurance and therefore operated through sick funds, and through the patient paying the doctor and claiming a refund. In Norway today all this is managed by a National Insurance Institution but the local offices, 740 of them, which is one for each commune, have considerable autonomy. A board of local people deals with local problems but the central body decides on the premiums to be collected, runs an equalisation fund which ensures the solvency of small local funds and generally supervises the system. The employed, the employer, the State and the municipality all contribute to the funds, those in employment contributing about half the total. The citizen who needs a doctor's care pays a fee and gets back from the sick fund a varying amount, as low as 60 per cent, as high as 100 per cent, depending on a scale of fees agreed between doctors and insurers. Many doctors are content to take only the scheduled fee and may therefore make a contract with the sick fund to be paid that amount and so save their patients the trouble of claiming, and making their own book-keeping much simpler. (Even then the doctor may ask the patient to pay a little direct to him for some services.) All other kinds of care, preventive, maternity, hospital treatments and admissions, are free to all. Occupational illness and injuries come under a separate insurance arrangement. Drugs may or may not be free depending on the disease and the type of prescription. For a very comprehensive service the average cost to those paying by weekly premiums is about 2.5 per cent of the income, around £24 a year. The patient has free choice of doctor but in remote areas that choice is limited, the doctor has to cover a very wide range of duties and techniques and his income is therefore guaranteed by the State. It is said that in these areas the individual doctor 'represents the national administration but is the servant of the people of his area'.

The Norwegian system covers mental disease and dental care, has special public health laboratories and its own system of pharmacies which are part public, part private. Norway is a small country and has had to strive deliberately to raise its standard of health care—indeed Dr Evang claims, 'Norway is not a country where the medical profession generally performs low quality work'. It is one of the European services which illustrate how well an organised service, publicly controlled and partly paid for by taxation, can work, and fully justifies Dr Evang's considered opinion that 'medical care has reached the highest level where prepaid medical systems are fully developed'.

The same can be said of Denmark, whose 5 million inhabitants are very well covered by services with a history going back to 1882, but now operated under an Act of 1960. What started as a voluntary system for some groups of workers is now 'universal with 96.7 per cent of the people actively insured against sickness'. The local insurance funds are now organized nationally so that the same rules apply to all, since all may be sick, and those who do not actively join are required to be associate members of a fund. There are a national scale of payments, incomes for health workers and fees for doctors. The system is somewhat complicated and even erratic but this is due to the long slow evolution, and the taking in over the years of different classes and groups. The medical profession played an important part in these developments and has many duties in today's administration.

We need not go into Denmark's service in every detail as it is already well documented, but it should be noted that while the insured contribute about 75 per cent of the cost of the general practioner service, hospitals are free and largely paid for from central taxation. Citizens are divided, on an income level laid down annually, into two groups who pay slightly different premiums, but can get largely the same service. The primary contact is a general practitioner and the specialist is paid for only if the family doctor has referred the case to him. The patient is free to choose his doctor, the method used in the country being a little different from that used in the capital, Copenhagen, and payment is by capitation fee plus other payments. Those who are in the upper income groups pay the doctor and claim a refund, as is the usual continental pattern. Hospitalization is free and unlimited in time. In theory the sick funds pay for every patient but as the cost of hospital care has escalated, the payment is no more than a token. The rest of Denmark's services, costs, attitudes and new developments are very like those of Norway and need not be detailed. The system is under constant review and seems likely to move forward to some kind of health centre service linked to hospitals, where specialists are already very largely salaried officers for whom private practice is not permitted. Ethically, indeed, the Danish specialist tends to look down on those who do private practice at all. The hospitals in Copenhagen are linked through a central bureau which controls admissions and makes most of the out-patient appointments so as to smooth out the daily load. There is a national system for prevention through hygienic measures, immunization and school health care. In many areas the family doctor, assisted by the usual team of health visitors, school nurses and midwives, does a great deal of this work. It can be said of Denmark, as of Norway, that a positive attitude to health is wanted in health and social security so that all Denmark's inhabitants can be assured of a good life.

As we go south from Scandinavia we find a little less insistence on the need for schemes covering 100 per cent of the people, and schemes are less straightforward but still in the same basic structure. The family doctor remains, he is paid by the patient who claims back from a sick fund to which he has contributed under a compulsory scheme for those below a certain income; and hospital care will usually be free but not organised in one service. In Holland, for example, health insurance is compulsory for about 70 per cent of the people but others, usually 10–15 per cent, join a sick fund and receive the same benefits. The remaining 15–20 per cent purchase private health insurance as their whole protection or combined with membership of a sick fund. The 115 sick funds are supervised by a central Sick Fund Council which collects premiums from employers and employees, plus a government grant to cover those who are too poor to pay or are aged. Because of their origin, which was largely in medical organizations, the sick funds are very much concerned with the quality of service, but they also try to control expense. Patients register with the doctor of their choice, if he has a contract with a sick fund, and he is then paid by capitation fee. He may have 3,000 sick fund members on his list but he is paid more for the first 2,000. There is an official drug list and all drugs on it are dispensed free. But the sick fund member must be registered with a pharmacist who gets a capitation fee plus payment for each prescription. It is of interest and importance that the Dutch call the family doctor a 'house doctor'. This makes it very clear who is the primary care physician and there is a sharp distinction between him and the hospital specialist. The sick fund pays for those patients referred to a specialist by the house doctor. Dutch hospitals are still owned individually, just over half by religious bodies (both Protestant and Roman Catholic). Non-teaching hospitals get paid by the sick funds but need to be subsidized, and the university hospitals are covered and largely paid for by the State.

What most people find so interesting about the health system in the Netherlands is its continued emphasis upon domiciliary and community services and upon the part to be played by voluntary organisations. Public education in health is continuous and aided by many special services, for example for sailors, and by a good occupational service in many factories. Midwifery is still very largely a home affair, 70 per cent of births taking place in the woman's own house. A large proportion of births are managed by the midwife but she usually has aid from one of the voluntary bodies, the Cross organizations, Protestant, Roman Catholic and non-denominational. The citizen contributes to these as a member and can call on them for help in the home when it is needed for maternity or sick nursing. Emphasis will undoubtedly continue to be on domiciliary services and a very strong College of General Practitioners, recognised by the State, is advocating the improvement of home care by organising the domiciliary team of family doctors, nurses and midwives through health centres. Laboratory and X-ray services, too, are now being made available at local hospitals for all who need them.

Neither the Scandinavian countries nor the Netherlands are very large. The problems of a health insurance system seem larger when one turns to France and Belgium with nearly 60 million inhabitants. They have developed their medical services along similar lines but it must be said that the medical professions in both have not been so helpful or forward looking as in the places already discussed. There have been almost inevitable arguments with the government about fees; for in an insurance claim-back system there has to be some standardisation of charges and this is always a problem.

A writer in *The Times* (16 July, 1971) described the Frenchman's attitude as 'a desire to have his cake and eat it', and said that nowhere is this more clearly illustrated 'than in his attitude to social security and national health'. The public want every kind of benefit and free choice but do not want to pay more in contributions. This he says applies equally to the doctors. 'Two enduring controversies illustrate this aspect of the French character. The first is between the social security service (which includes national health) and part of the medical profession over the Government's plans for a new national convention on charges and prescriptions for a period of four years.' The idea is to fix new fees 'to curb the alarming increase in expenditure' while preserving what the doctors call 'essential principles of liberal medicine'. There have been violent protests against any attempt to deal even with obvious excessive charges and over-prescribing.

We need not dwell on the second controversy, which is over whether self-employed and non-employed should pay more or less for their partial social security: but we may note that in France these citizens, the small farmer, the artisans and the small shopkeeper, represent a very much higher proportion of the population than in most European countries. They have also provided a good part of the private practice income of the French doctors. Fundamentally this is really an argument about how to finance a health service for all. The French are becoming more and more aware that an insurance system based on contributions from those covered plus a claim-back system which does not have a completely binding scale of fees will not satisfy everyone. Nearly 100 per cent of French people have cover: but the system remains very diverse and erratic and leads to this kind of argument every time a change in finance is needed.

In both Belgium and France development has been over a long period, interrupted by two world wars, and the French system is particularly complicated. The health care insurance now covers over 90 per cent of the total population, and everyone below a certain income. The insurance is part of the general social security system and those who have not paid contributions, the poor and the aged, are brought into the scheme by payments from general taxation. Some diseases, for example tuberculosis, are covered by special services, but otherwise the service is comprehensive and the contributions are graduated according to income and paid by both employer and employee.

The doctor of first contact is in these countries also the general practitioner who still works as an individual, and likes to fix his own fees in spite of the national schedule. But there are penalties for a doctor who is found charging more than his skill warrants. He does both office and home consultations but he has no fixed list of patients, and a patient may indeed go direct to the specialist. But this 'fee-for-service' system is not able to meet many needs, and so France has a chain of well over 700 publicly owned dispensaries for maternity, infant welfare and school health services, free dispensaries which are regionally or locally administered; the social insurance officers can use some of their money to extend into other fields, including alcholism, which is a great health problem in France. Mental health clinics are also provided and it is claimed that France aims at more than covering payments for certain health risks. She aims at prevention and the promotion of positive health.

France has a large provision of hospital beds, over half a million, and they may be publicly or privately owned and may indeed be profit-making. The public hospitals are variously controlled and the many religious institutions are largely giving a public service. Their income is derived from the individual patient but he in turn claims it from the social insurance funds (or social welfare if he is not insured). There is a move in France to reorganize the hospitals and bring them into some kind of planned and centrally controlled service. It is proposed that 'regional hospital centres' would be the main units, completely equipped, in a linked service of smaller places. These are however intended to be well equipped and well staffed. In many of France's largest hospitals the staff work on the 'firm' principle and all have full-time contracts: but up to 8 per cent of beds may also be available to senior consultants for fee-paying cases. The French hospitals, as in most countries, absorb the highest proportion of the total spending and the hospital is seen as the main unit of the disease treatment services. There is therefore some as yet unresolved tension between hospitals and the general practitioners among whom there is a move to build health centres and bring more work back into the community.

Of Belgium it need only be said that the pattern of health care follows the European style in most parts but with particular variation in the hospitals. Less than 40 per cent of hospital beds are in public institutions and Belgium has for years been trying to bring its hospitals under some kind of national plan. Since the insurance funds provide the biggest part of hospital incomes a good deal of indirect pressure was always possible, but many studies revealed how inefficient the use of beds was and how variable the standards of care. Children's care was considered especially neglected and in general terms there were more surgical beds then any other kind. Today the Ministry of Health, under a new law, has assumed ownership of all hopitals, so that planning becomes possible, but most have been left in the hands of the original controlling bodies for the day-to-day administration. It is thought that this and other developments will lead to more and more of the religious order hospitals passing to non-religious, probably public, bodies. Meantime the hospitals obtain most of their income by charging all patients a fixed charge per day, laid down by the Ministry of Health, of which the amount actually paid by the patient depends on the type of hospital. Patients in private hospitals usually get back 85 per cent but those in communal hospitals, whether insured or not, get all treatment free.

The general practitioner service is the usual fee-for-service scheme, the patient paying the doctor according to a negotiated scale of fees and recovering between 75 and 85 per cent from social insurance. Diagnostic aids, X-ray and so on are paid for by the insurance funds and the service may be given by doctors working at public or private hospitals. The whole question of fees is a continual source of disagreement in Belgium, disagreement between doctors and the insurance fund, that is the Government, with patients anxiously watching as the amount they have to pay may be quite a drain when they are sick and being paid probably only 60 per cent of their normal wage by the insurance fund. At the same time over 90 per cent of the people of Belgium are insured and today many argue that it would be more efficient and less costly to make the service comprehensive and convert it to a full national health service.

The European pattern reappears in other countries with local variations. Because it needs a large local and national bureaucracy it is more costly in non-clinical spending than a service which does not have the problems of claiming back money from a third party after paying the doctor. It can be seen that planning is less effective and this applies especially to hospital services which have often to be paid for or at least subsidized by the State. It is clear, too, that the mechanism of sick fund insurance cannot be applied to disease prevention, although some sick funds, as in France, do apply money to preventive services, but nowhere have they been applied to health education. But all the countries using this type of service are in a continuous ferment of change and most changes aim at getting away from insurance and separating entirely monetary payments for living from services for health.

Chapter 7

Some Other Countries

It is probably true that no country could today copy exactly what another country has done and certainly this has not happened, in spite of the strong resemblances between health care systems which have been brought out in earlier chapters. The historical fact is that medical care has been drawn into similar lines of development by the combination of scientific discoveries of the causes of disease, especially epidemic infections, and the fact that other scientific developments are life-saving only if enough money is spent on them. To overcome the epidemic diseases public interest and activity have to be roused and public money spent on clean water and food, new sewage systems and then mass immunization. To pay for the increasing cost of hospital equipment and staff, former poor-law and charity institutions had to be transferred to public ownership and while schemes of health insurance enlarged to include more and more people, hospital services needed to be subsidized by governments. At the same time reformers in every country were advancing political and ethical arguments as to why health care must become a community responsibility. This latter argument was finally accepted in the United Nations declaration that health and health care should be inalienable rights of every human being.

So we find that such diverse countries as Spain and Portugal under their forms of dictatorship, Turkey after its internal revolution, and parts of the British Commonwealth such as Australia and New Zealand, all had to introduce some kind of organized and State sponsored system. The less well-developed countries also found that they could not leave health care to private practice and slowly they have developed social insurance methods to include health care or have declared themselves in favour of a universally available system. These countries, however, are quite unable to produce a universally available system of modern medical care because their annual per capita income does not permit the building up of the necessary institutions or the training of staff. The prime necessity then becomes the conquest of epidemic disease whether it stems from bacterial or other infection, or poverty. In these efforts some aid has been given by more affluent societies and great efforts have often been made by individuals and by religious and charitable bodies. In some countries – in Africa, in India and in China – traditional forms of care have been kept in operation and have even become the subject of study and development. As with the developed countries already discussed medical care comes within the political field, for priorities in the face of poverty are usually more important than in a state of affluence, although even then decisions have to be made.

Spain, Portugal and Turkey stand mid-way, neither under-developed in the fullest sense nor fully modern and affluent. Indeed their annual per capita incomes are still low and all have a hinter-land, outside areas of industrial growth, where basic poverty is coupled with poor health care. Turkey has made an exceptional effort to meet this need, but still lacks the necessary resources and man power. Spain and Portugal, being close neighbours in philo-sophy as well as in geography and having similar health problems, have developed along somewhat similar lines. For centuries the Church played a large part in providing some hospital care but there is still a gross maldistribution of all medical services and the State is forced to take an increasing part in its provision and financing. The amount of money available is still not enough to provide modern health care for all, but both countries have in their cities hospitals and staff that compare with those in other European cities. It can be said that both countries now have a form of insurance for medical service as part of social insurance, with a large proportion of their people still getting at least hospital care in the same way as the poor have got it for centuries.

In Portugal the total money spent on medical care comes in part from premiums paid by workers and their employers, and in part from local municipalities and from central government sources. Public hospitals give free in-patient care to the majority of the people. Basically the general practitioner provides primary care at centres built and maintained by the insurance funds. Such doctors may be salaried or may obtain their income by a combination of a small fee paid by the patient plus a capitation fee and in many cases a payment for each item of service. The Social Insurance Institutes are very varied, some of community origin and others based on industries. Every trade and profession has its own insurance scheme and workers often have a joint arrangement between them-selves and their management. In a sense some of Portugal's schemes are the reverse of those in other countries, as it is the higher income groups who must be insured. The poor may get all their health care through communal services staffed by salaried doctors. It is claimed that one way or another most Portuguese can and do obtain their medical diagnoses and treatment from salaried physicians at hospital or health centre. The hospitals are organized, since 1962, by a Directorate General of Hospitals, and the State owns many of the largest hospitals but plans to have a chain of regional and local hospitals in the near future.

Although Portugal has general practitioners a very large proportion of primary care is still obtained through hospital out-patient departments. Very large numbers of patients are treated in emergency departments which accept not only casualties but all walk-in-cases. That this is not a service for minor ailments only is shown by the fact that 40 per cent of those asking for treatment are referred to senior specialists with a view to admission. All who walk in in this way are expected to make a contribution towards the cost, but it is claimed that nearly 80 per cent of the people get free treatment. The insurance fund makes its donation for every member who attends a hospital. Private practice may be carried on inside public hospitals but the accounts are rendered by the hospital and a proportion is deducted to cover, in particular, nursing costs.

As with most countries Portugal's hospitals are a mixture of very old and very new buildings, but equipment is modern and computers are now being installed, primarily for administration, though it is hoped to use them also for clinical research and other medical purposes. The profession would like things to move faster and complains that not enough is spent, and this is felt to be wrong since the State has accepted the right of every citizen to health as a matter of principle. The insurance system is growing and expanding and as more people come in more money will be available and the present slow progress may be greatly speeded.

Much the same could be said of Spain, but the general system of social security, which includes health, does not cover more than 60 per cent of the population. There is a National Institute of Social Security which comes under the control of the Ministry of Labour. Its funds are the usual mixture of premiums and additions from the State. Employers pay their share of the general premium plus an additional amount to cover industrial accidents and rehabilitation. The health care system in theory covers all forms of medical attention, in the home, in the clinic and in the hospital. Hospitals now come under a central commission which, following the world-wide trend, has the task of co-ordinating the hospitals by means of a regional plan which will take in both the old religious institutions and the modern buildings built in the past twenty years from social insurance moneys. The same funds have also built over 400 local clinics at which both general practitioners and specialists attend. House visits are numerous and the GP is paid according to the number of families on his list. If they do public health and preventive work, as most do, their income is augmented, as it is by some private practice. Spain has the usual shortage of doctors and some small clinics are staffed only by a nurse.

There is much discussion, and indeed activity, in Spain on how the hospital services, which is free to those who are poor, charged at a low rate to others and allows limited private practice, is to be reorganized. Coupled with this is the problem of medical education which is less practical than it should be because of the shortage of beds in teaching hospitals. Spain has traditionally given medical education to students from Latin America and this is an additional burden. All in all Spain illustrates that in modern times no matter what the basic philosophy and political structure of a country may be, if health is to be the right of every citizen, health care has to be organized and its finance guaranteed by the State.

That is also the lesson from Italy, which has had a Ministry of Health only since 1958 but is already trying to weld into one plan the half million hospital beds that serve its 50 million people. There were once a very large number of health insurance funds, but these are now amalgamated into a few large sick funds of which membership is compulsory for all employed persons. The contributions are salary-graded but the employed person pays much less than his employer. What is exceptional about Italy is that she has two distinct government supervised funds, one for general sickness care, including families, and one for industrial hazards and accidents. Both own hospitals and clinics, while other hospitals are owned by municipalities and by private organizations. The insurance funds have contracts with most hospitals. The National Institute for Sickness Insurance covers both medical and financial benefits but has a time limit of only 180 days, after which the patient who cannot pay (and those who have in any case not paid contributions) turn to Public Assistance for further help. This Institute has over 900 health stations and it is at and from these that the bulk of medical care is given. The size and staffing of these polyclincs are very varied, depending on population served and the availability of hospital beds and hospital specialists. Payment is by a variety of methods and all doctors, as a rule, carry on some private practice.

The Italian National Institute for Insurance against Industrial Accidents is unusual in many ways and has excellent staffs at its main hospitals. The funds come from the employers who pay a weekly scale for each worker, and the siting of the hospitals and clinics is, of course, related to industrial areas. In some cases a part of an existing municipal hospital may be used for this service. The staff are paid by salary, but many do additional hospital work elsewhere or see private patients with traumatic conditions who are not eligible to use the accident hospitals. The Italian approach to many health problems is through industry, probably because the Ministry of Health is not in control of the insurance funds which operate under the Ministry of Labour.

Anyone studying the problem of health care finds what is happening in Turkey exceedingly interesting. Turkey still has a very low per capita income and has many health hazards. It is a large country, more Asiatic than European, and any service has to be constructed in such a way that it can serve the rural eastern areas as well as densely populated Istanbul. This variation in population density and in wealth engenders the conditions that lead in all countries to maldistribution of doctors, and it is this question that is behind Turkish thinking on the subject. Turkey has settled for a health centre service in all areas, but capital expenditure has been concentrated in the rural areas, and doctors are paid higher salaries in the country than in the towns, where however private practice is still a financial magnet. With 31 million people, Turkey has a very low number of hospital beds, only 1.7 per 1,000 people in 1963, and not many added since. Nursing, in a Muslim country, was never recognized as a suitable profession for young women, and doctors are in very short supply although two new medical schools have been opened in the last five years.

Some ten years ago, Turkey decided that health must become a right of every citizen through a 'socialized service'. There was a form of health insurance but it covered a very small proportion of the people, and the poor, who are the majority, had to be provided for by a nationally operated and financed service. The country is now divided into 'socialized service areas', each of which has a health centre large enough for between 5,000 and 10,000 people. The staff should be a doctor, a nurse, a sanitarian, two or more midwives and a driver. The description is very like the feldsher post of the USSR except that a doctor heads each one. There are now over 300 health centres, 250 dispensaries and over 3,000 medical aid posts, some of them mobile. Every medical student has to spend some time at such a socialized unit and every graduate is expected to work in a rural area for some years before settling down to his permanent career. The full socialized post is, however, a number of such health centres grouped around a small hospital at which a small team of specialists work. In addition to their duties in the hospital they also visit the surrounding health centres.

This experimental service is already spreading all over the country and meantime there are a great variety of arrangements, especially in the cities. Although the system is supposed to be insurance based and patients, going to hospital, for example, should pay and claim back the money, in practice almost anyone gets free hospital care. The effect of this is that very large numbers attend hospital out-patient clinics and the university hospitals are particularly crowded. Specialists are salaried officers but are usually permitted limited private practice after their day's work at the hospital is finished. The university hospitals are owned and financed centrally; most hospitals are municipally owned and financed by the usual mixture of insurance, direct payments and local rates. It must not be thought that because so much of Turkey is still very poor the standards of the best hospitals fall below those further west in Europe: some of her institutions are fully geared to all aspects of modern medicine.

Another country with a low per capita income and innumerable health problems which has had to make decisions about health care is the subcontinent of India. In a country with over 520 million people where poverty and malnutrition have for centuries been accompanied by mass epidemics, health care is an absolute necessity, and on gaining independence India made it one of her priorities. The problems and the great efforts made to overcome them need to be seen to be understood, but the present writer had an unexcelled chance to do so. As the first Aneurin Bevan Fellow appointed by the Indian Government to tour the medical schools of the whole country, an attempt was made by him to assess the present position, and part of the story is told in *India: Which Century?* (Gollancz, 1967).

India has unfortunately the same problem with doctors as other countries—maldistribution. In spite of its overall poverty there is still great wealth in India, and half of India's doctors are to be found in the larger cities serving the wealthy; a devoted half of the profession works in the rural areas and smaller towns, usually on a not very adequate salary. One decision India has made is that she will try to educate enough doctors to provide a universal service and she has built, in just over twenty years, sixty-five new medical schools, each with its large hospital. But the outstanding fact about India is that 85 per cent of her people live in the country and there are some 700,000 villages. In the places where there is a large hospital its out-patient departments are daily overwhelmed by hundreds of really sick people. Many in India recognize that a hospital should be a place for special care and that ideally only those cases already referred by a physician should be seen. But this, in India, would necessitate many thousand more doctors, and it will be a long time before enough are trained.

Nevertheless India's future service will be based, like Turkey's, on health centre units in the villages staffed by the necessary team of doctors and other health workers. As long ago as 1944 a plan was set out by the Bhore Committee 'to provide everywhere an integrated curative and preventive service manned by whole-time salaried staff'. That committee could not foresee India's financial position and left to a future government 'to decide whether medical services should be given free to all, or on a system of payment by insurance or by some other method'. So far as the agricultural community is concerned it has to be a free service, but India is trying out State supervised insurance for industrial and governmental service personnel. In theory, and increasingly in practice, India's service will be based on a system of health areas or blocks and in each there will be, for some 40,000 people, a number of primary health centres grouped around a hospital of 30 to 40 beds. Such a unit, it is considered, needs a total staff of doctors, midwives, nurses, sanitarians and so on of 33, which is quite a viable unit. These blocks would at the next level be linked around a large hospital at the centre of one or two million people, which would have satellite secondary health centres, similar to the primary ones but larger and staffed by both specialists and general practitioners.

Progress depends on the twin factors of capital expenditure and training of doctors and health workers. India tries to work to five-year plans. Her aims are well set out in *Preventive and Social Medicine* by J. E. Park (1970). Already, however, India has well over 4,500 primary health centres which have to take over much more than was visualized until the larger regional and subregional units are built.

One exceedingly interesting point about India is that health care is part of a scheme for area development, education, sanitation (water and sewage) and local democratic control. In other countries health care is part of an overall social welfare programme which does not exist in India. Health is therefore bound to and part of local government service and as general education and literacy improve health education, which includes family planning, will be under local control and initiative.

Indian medicine, teaching hospitals, health centres, all began under British rule and it is within the accepted Western medical system that India is working and training her doctors and nurses. Her medical schools still work sufficiently close to British standards and methods for thousands of young Indian doctors to come annually to Britain for further specialist training. Research institutes in India, following the traditions of the British pioneers in malaria and epidemic research, are working on the same lines of thought and using the same techniques as in the UK and the USA. Yet India preserves, and modestly supports, the ancient and purely Indian system of ayurvedic medicine. This is not just folk methods of alleviating disease but a complete system, the principal concepts of which go back to the fourteenth century. There are schools of ayurvedic medicine where historical techniques are to some extent blended with western ideas and the would-be physician is given some training in hygiene, prevention by immunization and even the use of modern antibiotics. With some 40,000 ayurvedic practitioners spread over the countryside India cannot afford to abolish abruptly this ancient system; nor would it be possible. But the larger, more scientific and better trained team of modern doctors and nurses should through the health centres ultimately give India a nationally organized service for all, as Bhore predicted nearly thirty years ago. And in the meantime India has many interesting experiments going on, some sponsored by international bodies, others by local people. The Voluntary Health Services built up by Dr K. S. Sanjivi at what he calls 'mini health centres' are among the most promising.

It may be that China finds herself in a similar position to India in her retention of acupuncture as a method of treating some diseases, and the retention of a good deal of folk medicine in the remote countryside. But China's modern medical schools are based on the same ideas as those in Western countries, and were indeed started and inspired earlier this century by doctors from many countries, especially from Britain and America. The doctors who have worked in or recently visited China are able to say that technically Chinese medicine reaches high standards, and the spread of health care, universally available, through village health centres and stations is part of the overall strategy to rid China of epidemic disease. Health education aimed at positive health, as well as prevention, seems to be an important part of the medical system.

Throughout the world there is unrest in medical circles, and there are conflicts between the need of countries to have a first-class system of health care applicable to all citizens and the sometimes narrower interests of the medical profession. There are said to be two freedoms essential to the physician, clinical and financial. On clinical freedom there seems to be no quarrel anywhere in the modern world, although interference has been recorded and might be attempted under a dictatorship. Freedom for the physician to charge a patient directly is still seen by some as an essential part of the doctor-patient relationship, the idea being that even the sick value the care they get more highly if they pay for it personally. The idea breaks down under any ethical consideration, is seen to be impossible in low-income countries, is impossible in the fields of prevention and health education, and is no longer politically valid in an increasing number of countries. Whenever a country accepts that a citizen has a right to health the whole question of payments has to be dealt with. We may look at Australia as typical of the problems that arise between doctors and State when the ethical principles have not been classified.

Australia has a national health scheme which is an attempt to reach a compromise between the State's need and duty to provide health care and the profession's determination to remain in an essentially market-place position which it can exploit to the advantage of the individual doctor. As medical costs have risen in Australia as elsewhere the Government has had to take over part of the cost. This has been done by the system so much used in other countries of the patient paying the doctor and then claiming part, usually only half, back from the Government. But that half-fee can still be so high that many Australians take out private insurance policies to cover either hospital care alone or all their health risks. Those who cannot afford to insure usually cannot afford to pay the doctor. To begin with no attempt was made to standardize fees, but the Government found it was paying out more and more on reclaims and for some time has been trying to make doctors adhere to a list of fees based on 'the most common fee'. This is a very inexact definition and one to which doctors need not adhere. It is said that two-thirds of Australia's GPs have been charging more than the listed amount. Doctor's incomes appear to have risen sharply and the Government would now like to negotiate a lower and more binding list of fees.

This has heightened the political and ethical arguments in Australia and the Labour Party there has put forward new proposals. Medicine, unfortunately, would still be left in the market-place but insurance would be channelled through one nationalized organization and all citizens would pay 1.35 per cent of their taxable income to that organization. The Labour Party scheme would be a universal one, doctors' fees would be fixed (on a fee-for-service basis) and 85 per cent of the payment made by a patient would be refunded. Doctors who wanted a simpler system could send their account direct to the insurance fund. Hospital care and any associated medical fees would be met by the fund. For the citizen a full service would be guaranteed, for the doctor a satisfactory income coupled with full clinical freedom. The battle is, however, likely to be quite fierce in political terms and illustrates the situation which has arisen before and is bound to arise when the medical profession opposes instead of leading the fight for a comprehensive service. The story of health care to date has been that of the struggle to find the practical solution to the age-old problem of enabling the doctor to give every patient his finest and maximum care while ensuring the doctor his rightful financial and social position in society.

We shall complete this brief survey with a look at New Zealand, which has had a health service since 1938 and where discussions since then have been more on detail and on developments than on principle. New Zealand has a relatively prosperous population without such great extremes of poverty and wealth as exist in other countries, and this may have made it easier to find a system under which although payment is largely through taxation the patient still pays for some items and claims a refund. The service, derived as it is from British ideas of medical care, is based on the general practitioner who is now paid however on a fee-for-service basis. Over the years the GPs have increasingly ceased to inflict the necessity of claiming back money from the Government and have sent in their claim, based on the official list, direct to the Department of Health. The GP may, however, and very often does, ask for an extra payment from the patient. As elsewhere this is also changing as more and more the GPs leave solo practice and join partnerships, which do not include specialists. The GPs appear to be moving towards a health centre solution, for they make full use of nurses and health visitors who could better work from such centres. Only about 35 per cent of all New Zealand doctors, roughly 1 to 830 of the population of nearly 3 million, are specialists, and they are salaried officers of the public hospitals. Private practice is carried on in small privately owned units.

New Zealand has an excellent health record in all the usual statistics and has carried out some excellent experiments in child care, especially in the School Dental Service. It was from this service, much praised by dental observers, that the idea of the dental hygienist, a nurse specially trained to attend to children's teeth, spread throughout the world. This service, like hospital care, is free to the whole population, and so are drugs prescribed by the GPs. New Zealand has had the same experience as the UK. The health service introduced by a Labour Government has for a large part of its existence been controlled, through electoral changes, by a conservative party – the New Zealand Liberal Party may be so described – but the principle of government involvement in the provision of health care has never been questioned.

Patterns of health care, we may conclude, become very similar as governments take over more and more their organization, planning and finance; and the family doctor is still accepted by almost all countries as the ideal physician of first contact and as the man who can still best be health adviser and educator for his own patients. But the family doctors, or general practitioners, appear content, indeed anxious to join in teams for the better organization of their work. The team is however one in which those specialists in domiciliary services, a far more economic type of specialist than the hospital consultant (although he too must be in the team) need the help of all kinds of ancillary, paramedical personnel, and in many places the health centre is visualized as the place at and from which they can best carry out duties that are essential to every community.

It would appear, too, that the public go along with this idea. An American physician, Dr Max Seham, reported in an article in *Social Science and Medicine* (April 1969) on his visit to eleven countries, which included many we have mentioned here, and concluded that 'the majority of the people are enthusisastic about their health programmes'. Dr Seham thought this was largely because the practice of medicine had changed in modern times from being a competitive business to a social service. More and more studies of this nature are being undertaken and while some weakness and deficiency can be found in all the systems of care looked at, the overwhelming opinion is that organization, preferably on a national scale, is essential to the development of a high quality system of modern medical care.

We have dealt in an earlier chapter with the Soviet Union's universal health care system and it may be taken as the pattern which is followed in other communist countries in eastern Europe. However it must not be assumed that they are identical for the variations, within the general provision of health care for all, are as great as in the western European states. There is also a variation in the amount the communist countries spend on health, for all have not had the same rate of industrial growth. Romania is said to have built up its hospitals faster than others and has a fully integrated service in which diagnostic, curative and preventive services work very closely with the social services. As in all communist countries the national strategy is carried out and controlled by regional and local boards which are part of the overall administrative system. Romania uses and builds on a district physician who operates with ancillary workers from a dispensary serving up to 5,000 people. Not only are dispensaries linked together (if geography permits), but they are directly linked to the polyclinic and to the district hospitals. Emphasis is placed throughout the service on prevention and rehabilitation. Writing about east European countries in *British Hospital Journal* (22 May 1971), the hospital administrator T. W. Hurst said that his visits to several of them made him 'more and more convinced that the concept of positive health in these countries is worthy of more consideration by those concerned about the provision of an effective and economic health service'. From our brief survey of a variety of countries, under a variety of regimes, there would appear to be a great deal of that kind of consideration both needed and going on around the world.

Chapter 8

What Countries Spend on Health

It must already be clear that the cost of medical care has been a very important factor in persuading different countries as to the form of organization for the delivery of health care they should adopt. There are many interrelated factors in health care finance and comparisons are full of difficulties. Professor Brian Abel-Smith has suggested ways in which spending should in future be recorded so that worthwhile comparisons can be made, but other voices warn against too strict an effort to relate spending to clinical results. Dr Karl Evang in a passage quoted earlier weighs in against the doctor's being involved in these comparisons by 'The increasing tendency to ask the health administrator for proof that the health project which he is advocating should pay'. He does not believe that the money spent on health services 'should represent sound investment as judged by an economist'. He agrees, as all must, that the doctor has a duty to avoid unnecessary spending or extravagant and luxurious items, but declares that the 'health of an individual, as well as the health of the nation, cannot be measured in material terms'.

In the end each nation has to ask itself if it is getting value for the money spent. Within each system internal comparisons will often show up internal variations, some of which cannot be justified and many of which pin-point weaknesses in the service of a particular area. In the United Kingdom there is much more comparison, and much more is possible because finance is centrally provided and therefore well documented. When organizations like the European Economic Community are formed accurate figures become very important in attempting to reach common goals and common services.

Because of difficulties in getting together accurate figures many tables relate to periods such as 1961 or 1963, but a study of what other figures are available suggests that the ratio between countries remains much the same in spite of continued inflation and even devaluation by some countries. Baselines are often difficult to establish, some countries for example referring to their gross national product, some to gross national income and some to annual taxation income. The best study in the past ten years is that of Abel-Smith and Table 8.1 shows some of his figures for 1961. In Table 8.2 the same figures are used in relation to health expenditure,

Table 8.1 Spending on Health Care

Country	*Health spending as percentage of gross national product (1961 or nearest)*	*Per capita US $*
UK	4.0	57.5
France	4.2	69.8
Holland	4.5	54.4
USA	5.5	161.2

Table 8.2 Total Current Expenditure (1961 or nearest) including Services Paid for by Recipients, as Percentage of Gross National Product and National Income

Country		I *Total current health expenditure (millions)*	II *I as % of GNP*	III *I as % of national income*	*National income per head (US $)*
Canada	C$	2,045	5.5	7.3	1,475
USA	US$	29,859	5.5	6.8	2,306
Netherlands	G.	2,344	4.5	5.5	885
France	Fr.	16,374	4.2	5.5	1,079
UK	£	1,088	4.0	4.9	1,172
Sweden	Kr.	3,683	4.9	5.6	1,420
Yugoslavia	Din.	169,823	4.4	5.2	233

GNP, national income and actual per capita income. Yugoslavia is included in this table, although we have not discussed its type of national health service, because it illustrates that the per capita income is not necessarily the figure which guides the amount to be spent on health care. In countries with lower per capita incomes, India for example, a higher proportion of the GNP has to be spent if any service at all is to be provided. On the other hand Table 8.2

Table 8.3 Spending and Health Statistics

Country	*Percent of GNP spent*	*Crude death rate*	*Infant mortality*
Canada	5.5	7.7	27.2
USA	5.5	9.3	25.3
Sweden	4.9	9.8	15.8
Holland	4.5	7.6	17.0
France	4.2	10.8	25.6
UK	4.0	12.0	22.0

raises the question of whether the UK figure was at that time too low to provide the promised comprehensive service or whether it was a more efficient service than others. Attempts have been made to relate vital statistics to spending but a glance at Table 8.3, which gives some statistics for the same year as Tables 8.1 and 8.2, shows the difficulties. The UK crude death rate is high but is this due to faults in medical care or because we have an aged population? Holland has a lower infant mortality rate with a domiciliary service, but the UK rate is better than the USA where most births take place in hospital. It is probably better for each country to look at its figures over the years and try to assess what effect not only health care but also the general social change is having on vital statistics. There are still enormous social class and geographical differences in every country and these are a better guide to what has to be done than simple statistical comparisons between very different societies.

All countries try to make these internal comparisons but probably none publishes more detailed figures than Sweden. The National Board of Health there publishes many figures and issues an interesting summary, *Rupro*, each year as a running commentary on how Sweden's health care is developing. The gross spending in Sweden remains high, 5.5 per cent of the GNP, but *Rupro* notes that while this is still rising the increase is at a slower rate than formerly. The health care moneys add up to an annual expenditure of about £86 per inhabitant (1,060 kronor). Of the total cost of sickness insurance, that is health and monetary benefits, the State provides 34 per cent, but when sick benefit payments are omitted it is seen (Table 8.4)

Table 8.4 Sweden: Sources of Main Health Funds (1969) (in thousands of kronor. Some items omitted)

Object of Expenditure	*Total*	*Income from* *The State*	*Local authorities*	*Employees*	*Insured people*
Sickness	11,325,700	2,474,759	5,128,885	2,000,705	1,690,683
Sickness insurance	4,244,349	522,292	—	2,000,705	1,690,683
General health service, hospitals and midwifery	6,243,070	1,725,800	4,517,270	—	—
National dental service	267,030	13,610	253,420	—	—

that the cost is very much the affair of the municipalities and county councils. This is because the bulk of the cost of hospital care falls on the local authorities, who find around 70 per cent of the total. The central government contributes about 13 per cent and the insurance funds 7 per cent of the total, the remainder coming from a variety of sources. Dr Bror Rexed, the Director General of the National Board of Health and Welfare, has put the Swedish attitude to spending on health very clearly in a forecast for the 1970s: 'The Swedish society with the state and the county governments in co-operation, have purposefully and rationally *invested in an expansion of health and medical care*, which has corresponded with the desires of the citizens. We are not now faced by any crisis which might force us to strike out without any clear lines of action.' He gave some very interesting figures of how health care had developed continuously in Sweden over a century and more, and concluded that they must follow 'a clear plan and a continued expansion of those fields for which science shows us possibilities and in which the people want a continued expansion of care'.

One or two countries have made close studies of what is happening in other places, and the Federal Republic of Germany has collected many statistics on how many people are employed in different fields. Some of these figures appear in Table 3.4, but they are not backed up by financial consideration. Of the spending on Germany's own health service many details are given showing how many different funds, insurance, State, regions, charity and so on make up the total. The spending follows a familiar pattern, the insurance funds, the State directly and indirectly through social welfare, and a small proportion through private payments and private insurance. The total for the Federal Republic of Germany is high, nearly 9 per cent of the annual national income but only 3.7 per cent of the spending by the Republic; compared with 18.6 per cent for monetary benefits under social security.

Spending on health in every country has increased steadily since World War II, has increased in terms of the currency of the country, in terms of real values taking, say, 1950 as the base, and in terms of the proportion of the national income, taxation income or gross national product. In the USA, for example, 4.6 per cent of the GNP was spent in 1950, 5.9 per cent in 1965, 7.1 per cent in 1970 and 7.4 per cent in 1971. That is the most spectacular of increases, but the UK has gone up in the same years from around 3.6 per cent to 5.1 per cent. Sweden, as we have seen, increased at about the same rate but is now slowing down. If we include in social services items other than those concerned with health and welfare, for example community services like education, fire service, roads and, as has been suggested, public transport, then there must be a clear government policy as to how the taxation cake is to be divided. In most advanced countries there is a sharp division of opinion as to how much is to be spent on war preparations and defence efforts, and those who want better health services, to say nothing of those health workers who regard war as a form of aberration from health, think too much is spent on armaments and armed forces. If we take present spendings and allow for further medical advances it would certainly appear that not less than 5 per cent of the GNP is necessary to give a service at all, that 6 per cent, as in the USSR, is not too much, and over 7 per cent by the USA would only be excessive if waste and inefficiency could be identified and prevented.

The second aspect of health costs involves the question of how the money is collected. If a great deal of money has to be spent in collecting sick insurance, drug costs, hospital bed expenses, charges for those things not included free, keeping watch on those who must for a variety of reasons – poverty, old age, disability – be exempt from all payments, the total bureaucracy can be enormous. One of the expected but to many people surprising results of a service, as in the UK, in place of insurance, as elsewhere, is the remarkably low cost of administration. The central cost is under 1 per cent of the total national expenditure and in each section, regional and local, of the other services the proportion is also small. In the expenditure of the US there is the cost of the largest health care bureaucracy in the world, but few figures are available. Insurance costs a great deal and of the total expenditure for 1965 3.1 per cent was the figure for 'retentions by the health insurance organizations for operating expenses, additions to reserves and profits', all, of course, paid by the people paying the premiums. In simpler terms, 'nearly 20 cents of every dollar paid in premiums to private commercial health insurance companies was used for administrative expenses'.

The insurance companies actually paid out in benefits for group policies 87 per cent of the premiums, but only 56 per cent on individual policies (1968). The non-profit-making schemes have quite high administrative costs, 5.7 per cent for Blue Cross, which covers hospital costs, and 10.5 per cent for Blue Shield, which pays the fees of doctors. The large government scheme Medicare spent 5 per cent of its money on operating costs.

The way in which the money is collected is shown for some countries and the year 1961 in Table 8.5, which is given as in the World Health Organization survey except that the money paid in the UK as social insurance is shown under that heading and not as money received from recipients, which includes fees and private pay bed payments. The proportions in all the countries except Canada and the US remain almost the same ten years later. But spending in Canada is moving very rapidly to the two headings of Government

Table 8.5 Sources of Finances for Current Expenditure on Health Services (1961 or nearest)

Country		*Total (millions)*	*General government (millions)*		*Compulsory social insurance (millions)*		*Other agencies (millions)*		*Recipients (millions)*	
				%		%		%		%
Canada	C$	2,045	376	18.4	604	29.6	319	15.6	745	36.4
France	Fr.	16,374	2,456	15.0	10,981	67.1	1,218	7.4	1,719	10.5
Netherlands	G.	2,344	486	20.7	994	42.4	98	4.2	767	32.7
Sweden	Kr.	3.683	2,440	66.3	450	12.2	—	—	793	21.5
UK	£	1,088	922	84.7	120	11.0	9.6	0.9	36.4	3.4
USA	$	29,859	6,683	22.4	491	1.7	8,456	28.3	14,228	47.6

and Compulsory Social Insurance as the national health insurance scheme spreads and consolidates. In the US spending moves more and more into government and paragovernmental channels. In 1969 the US spent a total of $60.3 thousand million, of which $37.7 thousand million were still in the private sector and $22.6 thousand million in the public sector. Between 1960 and 1970 the amount spent publicly moved from $6.4 thousand million to at least $25 thousand million and at the same rate of change 50 per cent of all expenditure will shortly be by various governmental agencies.[1]

One is tempted to include much of American spending, on Blue Cross and Blue Shield which are mutual aid societies, not commercial insurance bodies, as quasi-government spending, were it not that in spite of repeated statements about 'all Americans' being covered, 36 million in 1968 had no hospital insurance at all. The National Center for Health Statistics says that in 1968, for example, 57.5 per cent of 'non-institutional' Americans had no insurance for visits, to doctors or home visits, 61 per cent had no cover for drugs and 97.5 per cent had no cover for any dental expenses whatsoever. In the US great emphasis is laid on laboratory tests and X-rays yet less than half of the people have any cover for these purposes.

There are probably only minor differences in how countries with advanced technical skill spend their health service money but much depends on whether any special problem attracts an extra amount of money. Table 8.6 attempts to put the spending of the UK and the US into one comparable set of figures, but different ways of keeping the accounts make it difficult to get an exact comparison. Capital expenditure on building new hospitals is not included in the UK accounts as published. It is now over £100 million a year

[1] Rice and Cooper in *Social Security Bulletin* (January 1972), gave the 1971 figure as 38 per cent of the total and 63 per cent was paid by third parties who actually paid 87 per cent of the hospital cost.

Table 8.6 Percentages of Total Spending in the USA and UK (1965)

	US[1]		*UK*
Hospitals	32.8		60.9
Physicians' fees	22.1		
	54.9		
		General medical	7.5
Drugs	11.7		11.2
Dental care	6.9	General dental	5.2
Spectacles	3.1	Supplementary ophthalmic	1.5
Nursing homes	3.2		
Medical research	3.7	not included	
Other	9.0		3.5
Construction	4.9	not included	
Government public health	2.6	Local authority public health	10.2

[1] US figures from Ruth S. Hanft in *Social Security Bulletin*, February 1967.

which would be a slightly higher percentage than is shown for the US. Hospital expenditute in the UK includes all salaries and wages whereas the American figures separate the incomes of all doctors. Nearly 18 per cent of the US figures are, however, for headings which do not occur in the British figures.

It would perhaps be better to look at spending in terms of what it costs to give whatever service is given to the citizen, and the World Health Organization survey gives figures for 1961 which are summarized in Table 8.7. These are in terms of per capita spending a

Table 8.7 Per Capita Spending in US Dollars 1961–2

Country	*Government and compulsory social insurance*	*Other*	*Direct*	*Total*
Canada	51.4	16.8	39.1	107.3
France	57.3	5.2	7.3	69.8
Holland	34.3	2.3	17.8	54.4
UK	48.7	0.5	8.3	57.5
USA	38.7	45.7	76.8	161.2
Sweden	73.7	—	20.2	93.9
Ceylon	2.8	0.2	1.8	4.8
Pakistan	0.3	0.1	0.7	1.1
Yugoslavia	11.0	0.9	0.8	12.7

year in US dollars and show the enormous range. However all these figures could be almost doubled to show 1972 spending which would not, however, alter the relationship. US spending per capita is now put at over $350 and the UK figure is $109. There do not appear to be any comparable figures for the USSR but *The System of Public Health Services in the USSR* 1967, shows that the expenditure for 'Public Health and Physical Culture from the *State* Budget' which was 3.12 thousand million roubles in 1955 had risen to 7.4 thousand million in 1967. However this does not include medical education, research or administration costs; and a great deal of money is spent by the trade unions, co-operatives and collective farms as well as local soviets on a variety of health activities. The USSR statistics concern themselves much more with details of hospitals, beds, clinics, doctors, nurses and so on, without giving the cost. The present five-year plan provides for still greater numbers of all these and other items. The USSR already has far more doctors than any other country and plans to double their number. The trade unions spend money on health services apart from the Ministry of Health, and in particular they pay for convalescent treatment at the many spas in southern Russia. This is regarded as essentially part of the health service but it does not show on the health service budget.

We have spoken mainly of health care cost in terms of the gross national product but many articles on the subject talk in terms of the national income. The USSR spends 6 per cent of its total budget which may represent some 9 per cent of the national income as calculated elsewhere. The Office of Health Economics has published its estimates in terms of national income as in Table 8.8. It warns

Table 8.8 Percentage of National Income Spent on Health Services (1968)

Canada	9.66%
USA	8.22%
Sweden	7.12%
France	6.56%
UK	6.02%

that these are estimates based on the original B. Abel-Smith survey of 1962, but they are of interest. The system in Canada appears expensive since it is not a service but an insurance system basically: but Canada has difficulties with vast territories and many areas of sparse population. She may be getting value for her 9.66 per cent of national income. The USA, one has already said, is not getting value for her 8.22 per cent. Edward Kennedy, addressing the Senate, said that the US was not getting value for what she spends and declared: '. . . from the day the Health Security system of national health insurance begins we will guarantee our citizens better value for their health dollar'. He went on: '. . . the comprehensive health services provided [by the new system which he proposes] will be available for the same cost we would have paid for the partial and inefficient services of the existing system'.

Of Sweden it can be said that her citizens get a truly comprehensive service of high quality; and she pays a little more for treatment in her excellent hospitals than she would if she had, like her neighbours Norway and Denmark, depended more on her general practitioners. France is exceedingly difficult to judge because of her diversity of service, but few people think she gets anything like a comprehensive service for all from what she spends as a nation. Great Britain cannot be judged strictly by comparison with any of these other countries because her system is a service, largely free therefore from bureaucratic costs but still not organized as her own legislation lays down; and she is still having to spend money on old, inefficient hospitals while she waits for new. But, as all the figures given here show, she gets her general medical service for a relatively low figure and can for very little extra put her quality of service ahead of most other countries.

Chapter 9

Problems for Study

A variety of problems have come to the surface in each of the previous chapters and the faults that have to be eradicated in any blueprint for future health care begin to show up. The problems of omission are many and the much more difficult question of visualizing future needs and society's future abilities has also to be tackled. One thing is clear: not only has the debate on health care begun, but all over the world the same problems arise and the same ideas and possible solutions are being discussed. Language, however, may present difficulties, for words used in health care discussions do not always have the same meaning. When we come to write about health centres, for example, we find that the British concept, dating from as long ago as 1913, of a place for the organization of a general practitioner team with ancillary workers, is not what is meant elsewhere. Sigerist, who did not use the term at all in *Man and Medicine* (1931), uses it with a variety of meanings in his book on medicine in the USSR published in 1937. Group practice similarly has a variety of meanings in different countries.

The discussions may be said to be of two quite different kinds. On the one hand there is the question of the type of system that is to be adopted and on the other the problem of control within the system, of trying to ensure the highest standard of clinical care and yet run the service efficiently, and to strike some kind of balance between a humane and personal service and an economic system which does not demand more than its share of the money available. As we have shown (Tables 8.1 and 8.2) there is considerable variation in what the developed countries spend on health care. When we look at Tables 9.1 and 16.1 we see that the amount of money available is very limited in many modern societies. Bryant in *Health and the Developing World* (1969) discusses not only the relatively small amounts on which some countries have to try to build a healthy population but also the fact that the problem is still likely to be there in AD 2,000, even if the gross national product is steadily pushed up by industrial development (Table 9.1 is from his Table

Table 9.1 Population and Per Capita Incomes 1965 and (projected) 2000

Country	*Population in millions*		*GNP (1965 value) Billions US$*		*Per capita GNP (1965 US$)*	
	1965	2000	1965	2000	1965	2000
Indonesia	105	239	10.4	29	99	123
Colombia	18.1	54.9	5.0	20	277	359
UK	55.0	60.0	98.5	389	1,804	6,530

10, modified). If the future holds the drawing together of the countries of the world and the lessening of international disputes, then health care will become increasingly a unifying force but it cannot be so if the present disparity in resources and abilities persists. So that while we may discuss the specification for health care for our own relatively affluent society, we must later return to the international problems.

One thing is no longer a problem about the National Health Service—it is here to stay. Already in 1962 the American Almont Lindsey could say, 'So much has it [the NHS] become a part of the British way of life, it is difficult for the average Englishman to imagine what it would be like without these services which have contributed so much to his physical and mental well-being.' The former Minister of Health, Enoch Powell, could write in 1966, 'The very contemplation of denationalizing the NHS is enough to daunt the stoutest political heart.' Six years later his equally Conservative successor, Sir Keith Joseph, was saying, 'We have a potentially superb National Health Service'. Addressing a meeting of the British Medical Association on 8 February 1972, he made it quite clear that the NHS was now accepted by his Party in spite of its earlier vehement opposition, and that his Government was 'giving a higher priority than any previous Government had given to the National Health Service and personal social services'. The Labour Party would contest that a higher priority is now being given to health than when the Labour Government introduced the service. The Labour Party is committed not only to the preservation but to the expansion and improvement of the service. We can assume that we need discuss only a growing and developing service but one based on the basic principles established by those who first put the subject into the Labour Party's programme and saw it onto the Statute Book.

The most fundamental of these principles is the separation of health as a service from all the rest of social service which remains basically a contributory service. Health is a right and health care is also a right to all who live in Britain, and has no reference to contributions to any fund. It is this separation which, as we have shown, marks it off from the insurance based systems, existing and proposed.

It is, of course, basic to some political philosophies that increasingly, as rights are recognized and agreed, where they involve finance they will be met from taxation, as indeed are many other items in modern society.

That question out of the way, the service still has to be given shape. Had the principles established for this purpose been fully carried out or had the political machine of British democracy looked like insisting on the principles, it might not be necessary to ask what lies ahead. The Act of 1946 laid down that 'it shall be the duty of the Minister of Health to promote the establishment of a comprehensive health service'. but no one has been able since to challenge any Minister in a legal way for failing to 'provide or secure effective services' except in a few cases where an officer has been found guilty of negligence. That phrase in clause 1 of the Act was expected to give citizens, individually or collectively, health workers and Members of Parliament and other bodies a really effective way of challenging the Minister. He has always been able to shelter behind some other person, the negligent employer, or a political position, most frequently lack of funds, or on occasion to deny even the validity of the words.

It is, at any rate, quite clear what kind of service was expected. It was to be universally available, it was to be comprehensive and it was to be 'free of charge'; and it is because two of these principles have not been observed that we now have to discuss and study them. The service is universal, but even that principle is broken by the existence of private practice within the service and by the attempt, even on the part of some Ministers, to extend it. Universality should have meant that every item of the service would be looked at to ensure that all citizens were getting the highest form of medical care 'free of charge' and that no encouragement or help was given to anyone who tried to give or to suggest that they could give, as individuals, better care within the service than the general standard permitted. It must be recognized that if a nation sets out to give a service to all its citizens it must have the aim to make the service the finest that can be organized. The position is different if the State is doing no more than offering to organize insurance or to subsidize existing services, for it can then think of itself as no more than an insurance agent selling a certain kind and amount of medical attention. But in a national service there can be no place for two standards of care.

Private practice in Britain is the chief element of market-place medical care that is left. There are certain health cults and there is a fairly large amount of self-medication which depends on buying advertised drugs, but these are outside the NHS. There has never been voiced in Britain any real objection to private practice outside the NHS. It is its inclusion within, which appears to give it official status and encouragement, which is fundamentally wrong. It is wrong on the political principles of the NHS, it is wrong in terms of medical ethics and it is wrong because it creates a small privileged class within the one million health workers who almost wholly do not have the privilege. The doctor who works full-time in the NHS is in many ways in a position of privilege and financial reward very different from that of other health workers; the man or woman who adds private practice is claiming a position denied to the great mass of his or her fellow workers. There are not more than 4,000 out of one million who, because the State has spent large sums on their training and because the State subsidizes them heavily, are able to use the resources and staff of the health facilities for their own gain. Because the patient pays a certain amount for a hospital bed per week, between £70.10 and £102.2 in 1970, it is overlooked that unless these beds were there, unless the nation had staffed and financed them, private practice could not use the 4,350 (England and Wales 1969) which are provided for the purpose. Included in the cost to the patient is a token sum of £3 per week to represent the capital spending now taking place; but at present-day prices it might cost over £20 million to build that number of beds with all the attendant equipment of a modern hospital. Then there is the anomaly, which an ethical profession would not permit, that the cost of the services of full-time staff in a hospital is also included in the daily cost, but on a basis of an average over very large numbers of cases, and with no figure included to represent what that full-timer might have charged had he too been in private practice. The difference is between pence and many pounds.

There is no increase in private practice in Britain and the number of private pay beds has dropped from 6,647 in 1949 to 4,350 in 1969. Nor has the bed occupancy improved over the years—it is a feature of private hospital practice that it can be lucrative only when there are empty beds to be sold to patients in a hurry which is not clinical. What has changed upwards is that the number of patients paid for by third parties has increased. Insurance against admittance to a private pay bed, and in its latest form with additional monetary payments, is now a fringe benefit, and the bulk of the increase in membership of such insurance funds is on a group basis paid for by business and manufacturing firms. It is another reflection on the kind of mixed economy in which we now live that an insurance company can make a profit out of illness and also out of the use of beds in buildings to the provision of which it has made no special contribution. (Its tax contribution is like that of any other firm.)

Private practice is not only contrary to the principles of a health service, it is divisory among staff. The not more than 4,000 doctors who do private practice (and for some it is a minor affair) have quite different incomes and claim quite different liberties from all the other 17,510 doctors and dentists on our hospital staffs; and very different terms from those given, for example, to the heads of blood transfusion depots who have a particularly responsible position in relation to human lives. It is surely no longer tenable in a national service that the man on emergency call to ensure that blood is available for a certain patient cannot get, and has never claimed, any payment other than his salary, while the surgeon who can operate only by virtue of the blood supplied can claim any fee he thinks the patient can and will pay. The only flaw in our otherwise unique blood transfusion service is that blood given freely by voluntary donors and processed and transported freely by the NHS should be used to enable an individual surgeon, already under contract to the hospital, to make a private profit. This raises an ethical point so large we must return to it later

Private practice within the National Health Service was an open bribe to consultants given by Aneurin Bevan to get them into the service. Bevan has said in his book *In Place of Fear* (1952) that he had pressed for the principle that 'the essence of a satisfactory health service is that the rich and the poor are treated alike, that poverty is not a disability and wealth is not advantaged'. At the time of his arguments with the medical profession, 1946–8, it seemed a small enough bribe that the consultants would come into the service if they had the use of just under 1 per cent of all the beds. (The low bed occupancy means that only one half of 1 per cent are so used.) But later he said, 'There can be no doubt that the privilege has been abused', and he went on to ask that 'the number of pay beds should be reduced until in course of time they are abolished'. If society is moving further from the eras of privilege this may happen by the withering away process: it should be a positive policy, for unless all health workers are employed as a united team much that is hoped for will fail to arrive.

When we come to discuss efficiency within the hospital service, and couple this with the need for better training for every young hospital doctor, it will become clear that having a large proportion of the senior medical consultants giving only part-time service to a hospital presents administrative difficulties and creates psychological dilemmas for other staff. Cases of real abuse may be rare but the atmosphere of a department in which the chief has clear interests in an aspect of his professional life quite divorced from his ordinary work is far from ideal.

Once a nation is committed to a universal health service it has to decide what the content of that service is to be, and the ideal can be far from what is realizable. Mention has been made of the great difficulty countries face when their per capita income is as low as in India, Turkey and most African states. Logically prevention might take first place, the young might seem to merit more care than the aged, the disabled less worth spending money on than the fit, and so on. In practice the doctor or the hospital finds that treatment of the obviously sick, those in pain and those injured makes a demand for care which cannot be denied. Basic medical care to cover acute conditions, therefore, appears always to have to be satisfied before real decisions on priorities can be made.

In Britain the decision was that the service was to be comprehensive. It was to be 'designed to secure improvement in the physical and mental well-being of the people of England and Wales and the prevention, diagnosis and treatment of illness'. However that is not even a very adequate summary of what comprehensive means: the definition of the word and of what should follow is the purpose of later chapters of this book. Because Britain has been able to provide a very wide range of services since the end of World War II she has done so largely by adding to what already existed rather than by preparing a plan for the next five, ten or fifteen years as other countries have done. Developments have taken place within existing services. Approaches to a really complete modern comprehensive range of care have been made only as pressures from outside the service have forced decisions on certain questions. This is a valuable and vital part of democracy; but it should not be an important part if we have a Ministry (or Department) of Health which has in front of it a comprehensive concept of the future. It must be part of the national strategy for health that the men and women responsible for it are ahead in their thinking and forward in their outlook, and it is they who should be indicating the priorities.

The third principle, that the service shall be 'free of charges', is more usually spoken of as 'free-at-the-time-of-use', so that no one should be under any misapprehension as to who pays for a national service. The nation pays, and wants value for money. But the really vital point is that not even the smallest barrier lies between the citizen and any item of health care. Those who firmly believe in the capitalist principles of the market-place or the Victorian concepts of self-help will still talk about people appreciating what they pay for, even if in the next breath they have to admit that millions cannot pay at all, millions could pay only a part and for most the expense of modern medicine could, as American experience shows, be a serious handicap and even financially crippling. There is in fact no valid argument along these lines, for our British democracy has spent the whole of this century moving away from such ideas. Even in industry, as we have seen in the decades round the middle of the century, there are innumerable cases where the nation has to undertake burdens, provide capital, give a variety of subsidies to bolster up essential but not completely self-supporting businesses. In health care we went through the poor-law provisions, the voluntary hospitals asking for charity in the streets, the backing of the general practitioners by health insurance, the municipalization of the hospitals, the provision of free immunization and the organization of a national blood transfusion service, to reach the national conclusion that none of these worked for the whole nation. We saw other nations trying to solve the problems of the growing cost of medicine by a variety of devices. And we finally decided at the election of 1945, when the issue was clearly presented, that all charges should be divorced from health care.

Unfortunately we weakened in our resolve and were led into a false position when it appeared that certain charges, beginning with prescriptions, would make some people appreciate their doctor's care better, would stop people abusing the service and would provide a lot of money that could be used for other things. All these arguments were without foundation. People's affection for their doctor does not depend on whether they pay a prescription charge or not; and in so far as the doctors were affected by this proposition they countered it by prescribing larger amounts of medicines so that their patients got value for money. There was no abuse to stop and every committee that has examined the question has said so. The sick are not in a position to abuse any item of the service, for their GP remains in charge and only doctors can order any form of care, treatment or diagnosis. If any doctors do not do this wisely they are least likely to be influenced by a charge on the patient.

As for large amounts of money, the total collected in 1969 was just over 38 million and this in no way influenced what money was going to be spent in that year or the next. NHS spending has been going up steadily each year as a result of inflation and of governmental decisions, and the estimated spending (at 1971 prices) for all governmental services is expected to increase at a rate of 2.7 per cent per annum. Health expenditure is expected to increase by 3.9 per cent, much more than any of the individual charges have produced and indeed more than prescriptions, spectacles and dental care are likely to provide. This way of collecting a proportion of the cost is quite irrelevant. The nation is going to spend at least £13,000 million between 1971 and 1976 and its economic strength will not be altered by adhering to its principle that health care must be free of charges.

The priorities must be discussed in depth for the decisions are far-reaching for the future. In the first place, are we firm in our decision that the citizen will normally obtain his primary medical care, whether preventive, diagnostic or curative, from a general practitioner? If so, we have to make many decisions about his plan and way of work, and his training. If his way of work is to be the focal point for the health team, do we adhere to our British type of health centre or do we move to a type of polyclinic? Is the GP's relation with the hospital service to be that of consumer of hospital care (acting for his own patients), or is it to be integrated with the hospital team by his having duties within the hospital service? Is he not, rather, to be the community care physician who uses all the other available experts for his community's benefit? If so, how do we select and educate our future GPs? From whatever strata of society they come they have to be given, should hopefully already possess, a sense of social responsibility. The GP, above all, must think of the patient as a whole and consider the service in its totality.

He will have a contribution to make which his predecessor, the single-handed practitioner, could not make to the control of the service. Can we achieve in our larger and more closely living population what Norway claims to have done in her remote communities—make the doctor the servant and friend of his patients, the adviser of his lay controllers and the guardian of the national strategy for health? He must be put in the right environment to do all this by the decisions we make about the administrative structure of the future. In doing so we must also make sure that everyone in the health team can make all these contributions too, and we must bring in the ultimate arbiter, the citizen, for health is and must remain the concern of the people.

Chapter 10

Democracy and Health

The term democracy, meaning government by the people or their chosen representatives, is used here in order to make it quite clear that it is the government of the health service with which we are concerned. A great deal of difficulty has been created by talk about management and administration in the service because the words are used by some writers—and the dictionaries agree—as if they had the same meaning, while other writers use them to refer to two distinct features of running a service. There is now a voluminous literature on the subject, including portions of two Green Papers and one white Consultative Document issued by three successive Secretaries of State for Health. All three confuse management and administration in a variety of situations where they are different, or fail to establish that they are one and the same. For our purpose it is the structure of the service which is important: within that the managers can get on with organizing and controlling the staff, and the administrators can see that policy settled democratically at any level is carried out, but using that amount of freedom and initiative which is permitted and essential to a service dealing with all the variables involved in providing services for millions of people through the skills of many hundreds of thousands.

In a speech already quoted the Secretary of State for Social Services, Sir Keith Josheph, told a medical meeting that while our health care standards are probably higher than in any other country, we have 'not yet found the ideal balance between local initiative and central financial control, nor the ideal linkage between the interdependent worlds of local government and health services; nor evolved in all cases a sufficiently dynamic and yet sensitive system of responding to the infinite range of needs of patients and their relatives'. One reason why these objectives have not been achieved is that the health services are administered by unrelated bodies which deal separately with hospitals, general medical services and the preventive services. It was a great weakness of the 1946 Act, and an unexpected weakness of Aneurin Bevan, that the NHS was not set up as one integrated whole with one administrative machine to run it. It can be said that each part of the tripartite control we have had for over twenty years may have done its own part quite well. But the deeper considerations of team work, of dealing with health questions as one question, of achieving the maximum co-operation and harmony, have all been impossible. Now it is agreed by all that in any restructuring the first decision to be made is that the service will be fully integrated under one chain of command.

There agreement ends, and we will largely ignore the great variety of suggestions that have been put forward because none of them begins by analysing what democratic control we need to cover the years 1970 to 2000, the kind of period we have to legislate for since Parliament does not like having to reconsider problems of this nature more often than once in twenty to twenty-five years. Local government is being altered and health schemes cannot ignore what is going on in that field, but all we would say is that what has so far been done in local government with the social services is so incomplete and meets with so little approval that we should feel free to consider health as a quite separate problem. It is certainly large enough to merit its own separate machinery. It will by 1975 spend at least £2,900 million or £3,000 million; it will employ well over one million people, many highly skilled and expensively trained; it will own buildings and land worth as much as the assets of any other institution in the country; and it will give hundreds of millions of treatments to a large proportion of the population each year. It will be expected to do all this as well as possible for the least populated areas of Britain and for the cities, and to do it all in the public eye and under the scrutiny of Parliament and ombudsman. It will have to do it in the presence of a scientific profession on which it will be spending a lot of money in developing new treatments for disease, and it has therefore to be flexible both in attitude and in finance. All this has to be done, if present Treasury procedures persist, under a financial system based on annual estimates submitted to and authorized by Parliament. It may now be suggested that if it works it must be in spite of such a system rather than because of it.

It has been said that democracy can be served by a centralized system, by submitting matters to Parliament and then controlling what is done centrally. This view has never found favour in British political discussions. It is very easy to devise a central managerial system which can be very similar to the corporate state of fascist type. Writing in 1942, in *Health for All*, the present author summarized opinion of that date as follows: 'There is therefore no suggestion of a State medical service which would be run from Whitehall.' Such a system 'would inevitably be too bureaucratic to have any chance of survival in what we hope will be a truly democratic post-war world'. It was somewhat tragic that the opposition to an integrated service which Bevan came up against resulted in administration's being 'frozen by the politicians [of the BMA and local authorities in particular] in 1946', as Professor J. N. Morris puts it in *The NHS: Three Views* (Fabian Society, 1970). He goes on to say that it was already out of date then, and has been incredibly static since, despite the transformations in health and care—and, one might add, despite the increasing development of new ideas of participation in control and very great pressure for new forms of public control. No one who agrees to an integrated service suggests a centrally controlled one. But it must be recognized, and the system must allow for the fact, that a national service paid for by central funds must have an element of central supervision. In the 1946 administrative structure the various bodies appointed are agents of the Minister, their liberty may be circumscribed by orders and instructions from the Ministry and they are always restrained by the budgetary system. Much pressure has been exerted, by regional hospital boards in particular, to allow budgeting over a longer period than one year and the carrying over from one year to the next of any unspent money. A certain amount of liberalization of budgeting has developed and as we have noted the Secretary of State himself now gives forecast budgets for five years. But the most economically minded board or committee is still unable to make savings in one year pay for new developments in the next.

In saying that there is no agreement beyond the principle of full integration we must not overlook the large body of opinion which holds that the structure must be a three-tiered one. The disagreement is on the position, membership and duties of the bodies to be inserted at each level. There are some who have advocated only one body below the Department of Health, but this on even the briefest examination is seen to be too removed from our ideas of democracy to be acceptable. Within a three-tier structure however there are so many ways of selecting, appointing or electing people to operate it that we must first be clear what we are trying to do, and we must find the method which Sir Keith Joseph (in the speech already quoted) agrees we have not yet found. We have not found it because we have not decided what democracy, control by the people for the people, means in health care.

It is easiest to begin this consideration at the grass roots, at the lowest level nearest the people. The Department of Health, we can agree, must be at the centre, must be responsible to Parliament and must have whatever powers and duties are needed to create a national strategy, but we do not need to define it further. But health care is a personal service, can indeed be a matter of life and death, and the people as citizens and as patients must be involved in it. As Dr Peter Draper and his colleague G. Grenholm have said (*Community Medicine*, 21 January, 1972), 'Unless the opportunities are increased for public involvement in deciding what the health problems really are, how they should be tackled (including how much money they should have), and how satisfactorily services operate, the NHS can be expected to continue to experience serious problems in adapting to its changing environment.' It is surely the question of 'how satisfactorily services operate' that is vital to the people, and therefore their representation must be at a level and on a size and type of committee which will be sensitive to the needs of its own community. At present the public has little opportunity or possibility of influencing the committees of the NHS, especially those concerned with GPs and hospitals; but it is not enough to try to produce a method whereby the people 'can influence' a committee appointed by someone else, as has been the case up to the present. It was just remotely possible to regard the administration of a hospital as a technical and managerial matter but this will not do for an integrated service. In the concept of team work for health the patient is a member of the team. His personal co-operation and understanding in his own illness or in the pursuit of his own fitness are vital to the success of the team. His collective interest is equally important, especially in view of the innumerable variables involved. Grenholm and Draper have put it very well: 'There is a pressing requirement in health care systems to cope with the variability and uniqueness that characterizes the consumer, whether the recipient is an individual patient, a neighbourhood or a region.'

In that last phrase lies the essential principle on which a democratic service can be built. The individual as patient must have the highest forms of medical care possible but clearly we cannot organize a service on that basis. It is the neighbourhood, the community, the recognizable entity within the demographic and geographic factors of the UK, which must supply and influence the basic controlling body. It can only do this properly through the correct democratic process of election. We once had local bodies, the Boards of Guardians, to look after the poor and their health. We now need a more modern elected group of guardians of our health, and it is here we should start our thinking on the subject. We have been continuously led astray by governmental, civil service inspired documents on managerial systems, on individual influence on appointed bodies. We must build the NHS on a basic structure which gives the people a voice so that they can avoid, and will be determined to avoid, the terrible scandals of Ely, Farleigh and Whittingham mental hospitals, because these and all the other health facilities are the places they and their families use.

At once the questions of what size, and controlling what kind of area, what unit of population and so on, are raised. All the suggestion that have been put forward have been wrong because they have tried to fit in with local government boundaries or tidy, centrally conceived schemes. The new structure must be functional even if it is untidy; and it need not conform to any existing boundaries. It has been repeatedly said, by the present Secretary of State among others, that there are no boundaries in the health service. Patients must be taken to the service they require, near or far, no matter which area they are in for other purposes. But in addition an integrated health service is going to be a big job and its basic unit is going to be quite large enough for an elected committee to control. Suppose we use 250,000 people as our yardstick for purposes of illustration. Such a unit will have 2,500 hospital beds in 5 to 10 units. It will have at least 5,500 employees. It will have 15 or more health centres, the whole of preventive medicine, the school medical service and the new occupational health service to look after. It will spend up to £15 million each year and have some control over research. It will have a domiciliary service of nurses and health visitors and its medical specialists will do at least 2,000 domiciliary visits a year. It may be involved in building a new hospital at a cost of many millions of pounds and will have to control the rebuilding and modernization of its existing buildings. Its staff will be doing a socially important job and will have to supply information about the health of the community to central organizations, determining what will be planned in the future. And throughout all this it will have to remember it is not dealing with nuts and bolts and lines of production, but with individuals and individuals in that most difficult state when they are unwell, disturbed or even dying. Nor will this work be done in a stable environment, for not only is there rapid technological change, but professional definitions and public expectations of care itself are also changing rapidly.

We have suggested taking 250,000 people as a theoretical yardstick and as we see it measures up to a size of organization which would need very good officers, would employ medical specialists of the highest standing and would require public representations to be knowledgeable and watchful. But the figure of a quarter of a million is one that is to be found in the literature on the organization of health care throughout the past thirty years and in all countries. Many studies have come round to some such figure as the ideal; and if we look at the literature on neighbourhood units, on the size of new towns with their hinterlands, and if we look at the present distribution of populations in this country, we will find that the most frequently nominated figure for organizing services is of the order of 100,000 to 250,000.

But we have already in the hospital service a concept which falls into a similar pattern, the district general hospital. When this was first suggested in 1937 in *The Walton Plan for a National Medical Service* the authors took the convenient figures of 100,000 people and 1,000 hospital beds as the unit around which a comprehensive service could be built. (The Walton Plan was so named from its origin among the staff of the Walton Hospital, Liverpool, a city which today has 1,070 beds for 100,000.) The district general hospital is now the accepted focus of hospital care in any community and by 1975 we shall have 170 newly built or nearly completed in England and Wales, of such sizes that each, with smaller satellite hospitals and probably a mental hospital, will serve a unit of 200,000 people. Many who now accept, indeed boast of the District General Hospital as an outstanding feature of our service forget that the idea was worked out in great detail by its originators, especially the late Dr H. H. MacWilliam, not only as a suitable hospital but as part of a suitable health care unit for a given size of community. There is no argument advanced in any official document as to why we should not use the natural catchment area of a district general hospital as the unit for a district health committee, which would be elected and would be responsible for the day-to-day running of the service within the national plan. Had it been proposed that new local authorities should be the bodies to control the integrated service then clearly boundaries would have been set out to fit that plan. But everyone asks for a new and separate type of authority to control health care, to advance the concept of community medicine, and there is no valid reason why that authority should not have its own simple boundaries (for these are not to be barriers) based on the size of the area the district general hospital would serve. There will be places where geography may suggest that two could be combined, but the total population should not exceed 250,000 and wherever possible a town should be joined to its adjacent rural area. Flexibility is essential and some existing arrangements which may exceed that figure could, if not too large, be allowed to continue.

There is one serious objection to having any unit too large, namely, that it would be difficult for members and officers to regard the service as a whole, one of the purposes of integration. Inevitably the district health committee, if too large, would divide up its work, and we would have a hospital subcommittee and others for general practice and preventive medicine—back almost to the tripartite service that has existed since 1945. The division of work among subcommittees is a feature of many administrative bodies, but in setting up a new form of control we should be able to select a size of unit in which the committee of an integrated service should itself, as far as possible, remain integrated. Other schemes are now being discussed, under which the numbers of local health committees would be cut down to some eighty for the whole country. They would be known as area health boards, and would each look after well over half a million people, in some cases many more. This would inevitably lead to the divison of work in the very way we are trying to avoid.

But more seriously they would not permit that sensitivity to local feelings and needs which is essential to a human and humane service. There are still inequalities in resources within the NHS. Some of these have strange historical origins and must be ironed out; but there are also considerable differences in local needs. Professor J. N. Morris in the Fabian Society pamphlet already quoted from (*The NHS: Three Views*) gives some very good examples. 'Swansea, Wallasey and Halifax with highest mortality from coronary thrombosis have the highest claim on intensive care units; the towns of Lancashire, with their lead in bronchitis, deserve the liveliest clean air programmes; further support should be given to retirement areas in the south east and around the coasts, and so on.' Part of the sensitivity to such needs must come from the medical workers and their staffs. But enlightened public support is essential and social problems with a medical aspect are more likely to be brought to the surface by ordinary people.

The tendency in modern discussions to talk as if it would be enough to have locally some kind of advisory health council, leaving the running of the service to people chosen for their managerial skill, is contrary to all democratic ideals in Britain. It is better to run the risk inherent in local elections that some unsuitable people will be elected, than to give the power of forming these committees to officials, as has been done with hospital boards and committees. The people of Britain want their health service to go on expanding and improving and they must be given the chance of electing their district health committees.

There is one difficulty in formulating a district health unit of between one and two thousand hospital beds integrated with ten to twenty health centres: there are some services, especially those depending on very expensive equipment or rare professional skills, which cannot be provided in every district or even in the larger areas proposed in some plans. Coupled with this is the question of the medical teaching hospitals which may be district general hospitals in one sense but have special duties in medical education. It was recognized in the preliminary writings on the NHS that many hospitals would be given in addition to their ordinary services some special duty for a highly specialized function; and that some places might be provided, as indeed they have been in the existing service, which would have no ordinary medical responsibilities but would perform a highly skilled service for a very wide, even national, area. There was therefore general agreement that this kind of planning and provison must be done either centrally or, as appeared best and was in fact the decision, on a regional basis. It was from this angle that regional hospital boards were created, and all plans for an integrated service recognize that regional planning must continue. Indeed there are services arising from domiciliary care, special disabilities in young and old, that under regional planning might produce services we have not yet had. But in recognizing the need for regional planning the three governmental papers that have appeared in recent years all differ as to duties, membership, method of appointment, representation of special interests and so on.

They disagree, and reach no very good solution, because they have not settled how much of regional planning is to take work away from the Department of Health and instil into it some local and regional knowledge, and how much of it is to control local units and committees and compel them to fit into a regional and national plan. It appears impossible for civil servants who advise on these matters to make up their minds whether they are planning for a democratic service or a corporate state. They lean towards the latter with vague phrases about finding the right people with the right managerial skills to form some kind of regional board but still hesitate to make it a really executive body. Managerial skills have little if any relevance, except in advisory or planning bodies. It is here that the widest possible administrative views and skills must be available tempered, and watched on behalf of the sick, by the knowledge and skill of people elected by the people or appointed to represent essential special groups which might otherwise be overlooked. Yet regional bodies are very difficult to appoint by any kind of effective election because of the area they must cover, say one-fourteenth of the country.

So it would satisfy our democratic principles if our regional health planning boards were representational and at least half of their members came upwards from those elected to district health committees, whose main services are, after all, to be the subject of regional planning. It is at this level that the control of the Secretary of State and the lead he wishes to give can be made effective by ensuring that he appoints, directly for his own purposes and indirectly from nominations from other bodies, the other half of the board. It would be for him to decide what special interests had to be represented, but clearly these would include medical education, the education of other health workers, the rights of trade unions, both those concerned with health workers and those concerned with industry, industrial groups, since occupational health must be watched, and so on. The chain of control over finance and the realization of the national strategy would meet at this regional level, leaving the district committees very free to get on with the day-to-day work and to do so in the public eye and always in the eye of the local and national press. Secrecy has no place in a public service which affects every citizen.

This raises the double-edged question of staff representation on the controlling bodies at both levels. There should be no secrecy over any aspect of the service where staff are concerned. It is regrettable that in its life so far there has been an almost complete failure to provide information to the health service staff except so far as it is given to the public. Only the medical staff, and many of them also complain, have had anything like open access to information as to what is going on in the service. It is implicit in early statements on the functioning of the health service that staffs have the right both to be elected to committees and boards and to form and have recognized advisory committees. The early days of the service produced many innovations which have not all been fully developed. It was recognized, probably for the first time in public service, that an employee could also be a member of any committee, even if he was a full-time salaried officer. Thus Bevan appointed men to sit on the board which employed them, or the hospital management committee to which they gave service; and it was very regrettabls that this was not carried to its logical conclusion that any employee could be so appointed, for it was almost entirely confined to medical men and women.

The debate was then, and still is, whether health workers should be eligible on a personal basis or as representatives to be members of district or regional committees, and whether health workers should be able to act collectively, by committee, as advisers to the bodies controlling the service. It was implicit from the start that, so far as hospitals were concerned, if a group of workers formed a committee which was constitutionally valid, it would be recognized as a body which could give advice. Only the medical profession saw this through and in every hospital group quickly established medical advisory committees which were then recognized. But they went further and secured more than the 1946 Act actually provided, a number of seats on every board and hospital management committee. Regional hospital boards found that, although some doctors clearly had axes to grind, the system of having medical members of their staffs on the board itself and also having a medical advisory body worked in practice. Since local executive councils had half their members drawn from the professions this did not arise in their case. Health committees set up by the local authorities often co-opted medical men but they were usually from outside their own service. Now a new situation arises, for in an integrated service it may be thought correct that all health workers should have the same right either to sit on or to be represented on committees or on advisory committees. The whole question of 'worker participation', which has long been such a thorny political question and is today very much under debate, has to be settled whatever the structure of the new administrative machine. If the lower tier is elected then health workers will not be members unless they stand as candidates for a political party. This they must be permitted to do. The elected body must seek its advice from properly constituted advisory committees. It must always be proper for a group of workers to set up its own committee and to proffer advice. But should there also be an advisory committee of representatives of all health workers elected by ballot? And should all health workers be able to vote not only for their fellow professionals but for all those standing for election? If committees and boards are appointed and democratic elective bodies are given no place in the integrated service, then some places on every controlling body must be given to health workers and nurses, technicians and all other grades must have the same rights as the doctors have hitherto had.

All of this may be modified in its operation if some kind of medical administration is restored or continued in the integrated service. In the past, two medical officers, the Medical Officer of Health in the public sector and the Medical Superintendent in the hospitals, acted in part as advisers, in part as executive officers. The regional hospital boards installed a new senior administrative medical officer and his work within a region and contribution to its planning have often been quite outstanding. But hospital medical executives have almost disappeared for lack of clarification as to their duties and new schemes, those of the Cogwheel Report, have introduced a bevy of non-executive medical administrators whose function, tenuous as it is, will almost certainly disappear in an integrated service. Most countries find it essential to have a Medical Executive Officer and the original idea of a triumvirate, the Group Hospital Secretary, the Group Nursing Officer and the Group Medical Officer has never been properly established.

In an integrated service the problems of who are to be the chief officers have to be settled, their duties defined and in the case of a medical co-ordinator (as he should properly be called) his status established. He should be a full consultant and have clinical duties but he should be paid more, not less, for doing the medical administration. Some of the disastrous revelations about hospitals which we have had in recent years make it obvious that a medical administrator must have wide powers and authority. But he must also have a duty to see that what medical skill and talent are available in his area are properly applied in the service of all. This could be the most challenging post that the doctor of the future can hold. He cannot, and indeed must not be the 1984 Big Brother type of figure which has been feared and ridiculed. If he is to guide a health unit to do its best for the whole community he must be a man of wide knowledge and compassion and must be given adequate powers; and he is another reason why a district health committee must not serve too large a population, for the medical man in charge must be able to supervise it all. Working closely with the socially minded doctors of the health centres he will be expected to inspire them to provide an ever-improving service and to ensure that the consultants are ready to aid the general practitioners in service to the community.

Chapter 11

In-Hospital Care

One of the side-tracking aspects of our health care system up to the present is the question of the position of the hospital in modern times. One thing is clear to anyone who takes a backward look: our hospitals appeared in a most haphazard way and it was not until the whole subject of a national health service was already under discussion that any question of organizing and co-ordinating the hospitals was raised. There were two stimuli to a hospital plan, the municipalization of the old poor-law hospitals in 1930, and the outbreak of World War II. But all the authorities did was to take groups of hospitals as they existed and try to use them in a planned way. But even during World War II it was a partial plan and was mainly concerned with using hospitals to deal with people injured in air raids and only incidentally to draw the hospitals together and try to use their beds in a collective fashion. None of what was done went down to basic principles and asked what kind of hospitals we need, where we need to have them and how they could make their maximum contribution to an overall health service. The setting up of a tripartite health service which separated general practitioners and hospitals and managed them in quite different ways has not led to any fundamental thinking, but rather to a host of ad hoc decisions. It says much for the principles of the NHS and for the great improvement and increase in consultant services that the hospitals have advanced even in the absence of a well-devised integrated plan. Professor Maurice Kogan in *The NHS: Three Views* says, 'The NHS and the hospitals within it have done remarkably well. No other country delivers hospital treatment to such a wide range of people, at so little cost, both financial and psychological'. They have done so with comparatively little in the way of absolutely new hospitals in new places but rather by improving, in some cases rebuilding, old hospitals and overall in increasing the number of staff and utilizing the facilities, especially beds, to greater advantage. In Table 11.1 the changes in utilization over ten years indicate what this has meant in patient service. Table 11.2 shows that it has been

Table 11.1 The Ten-Year Increases in Britain

	1959	*1969*
Population	50,548,000	54,023,000
No. of hospital beds	548,676	528,917
No. of in-patients treated	4,544,000	5,975,000
Average length of stay in acute beds	15.6 days	11.1 days
No. of discharges and deaths from available bed per year	18.2	24.6
Total out-patient attendances	48,746,000	54,944,000
Hospital staff (England and Wales)	470,621	613,285

Table 11.2 How Hospital Staff has Grown (England and Wales)

	1949	*1969*
Doctors and dentists (as whole-time)	11,940	22,724
Professional and technical (as whole-time)	12,518	33,245
Nurses and midwives		
whole-time	125,752	188,639
part-time	23,060	90,604
Maintenance and domestic whole-time and part-time	156,586	157,663
Administrative and clerical (as whole-time)	23,787	43,328

achieved mainly by increases in staff. Because there are still some shortages many people fail to recognize how the manpower has gone up in twenty years and why the hospital wage and salary bill accounts for over 60 per cent of the total cost.

We have written in the previous chapter as if the concept of the district general hospital is accepted by everyone and it probably is, but with reservation on many aspects of hospital care which have remained subjects of quite violent discussion. They are numerous—hospital care for the elderly, for the mentally retarded, the physically disabled, and so on. But there is also the question of whether we need general-practitioner hospitals, post-operative units, small cottage hospitals, etc. There is, for example, an Association of General Practitioner Hospitals, set up to try to ensure that small hospitals are retained in the NHS. The chairman of that body, Dr M. Emrys-Roberts, has said (*The Lancet*, 2 October 1971) that 'with hospital planning so dominated by the district hospital concept the future of the much smaller general-practitioner hospitals has been in doubt'. In Britain hundreds of small voluntary hospitals were built in the early part of the twentieth century and as we have described were staffed by local doctors, almost entirely GPs, until the profession itself moved away from this idea and specialists were increasingly invited to do honorary work at these places. It was for this historical reason that so many of the private pay beds were and still are in smaller hospitals. The regional hospital boards who took over all the hospitals soon found that in terms of utilization many of these places were inefficient and some were even dangerous, especially in surgical matters. So, as plans were made, the function of many small units was changed and the general practitioner, who has no contract of service with the hospital authorities, might have ceased to work within these buildings. But from the start this was seen to be wrong in places removed from any possible district general hospital, and wrong in places where GPs were prepared to carry out work 'within their own competence' in hospital beds. Many GP units were retained, and indeed some new ones created. Dr Emrys-Roberts in his article reviewed 400 hospitals in England and Wales, ranging from 11 to 70 beds, which still have partly or wholly GP staff. While planning of what he calls 'the rigid concept of the all-embracing district hospital' has gone on there has been some retention of smaller units for a great variety of purposes.

The earlier developers of the idea of the district general hospital were never in any doubt that this would be so. They spoke always of the district general hospital and 'its satellite smaller units', and always insisted that planning must accept that either the service would be taken to the patient or the patient taken to the service, whichever was in the patient's best interest.

But the separation of the GP and the hospital services, and above all the fact that the executive councils had no planning powers, has made rational consideration of this problem difficult. Because GPs and specialists are employed and paid by two entirely and unrelated methods, and there is still competition for such private practice as remains, proper planning is difficult. An integrated service and the inevitable and desirable salaried service in which there is no private practice will enable realistic planning to begin. Dr Emrys-Roberts in his article made a suggestion which will be feasible only when we have a united medical team and only if our local administrative unit is of the right size. 'Would it not be better,' he asked, 'to plan first at local level, to provide a service for each community to care for its own sick to the limits of its ability, and to plan for what is left, for all that is more complex in the district hospital?' He visualizes that so much could be done in the smaller units that the district general hospital would not need to be so large.

In fact there is probably an optimum size for a general hospital, one which requires and justifies a great deal of modern diagnostic equipment; which is economic in terms of all the non-clinical services such as heating, lighting, kitchens, sterile services; and which is efficient in terms of staff, for the major specialties must have more than one full team available, preferably no fewer than three if all emergencies are to be covered easily. There is without doubt a size below which hospitals, even those doing only restricted work, become inefficient and uneconomic, especially in bed use. One factor which certainly alters the situation is the great drop in the average length of stay in our hospitals. Modern surgeons like to get their patients up and moving as soon as possible after an operation, whereas at one time the post-surgical case convalesced in the acute ward, sometimes for up to ten days. There is a great deal to be said for having in each locality units which can take such cases and which can be supervised by the GP, but the number is not large enough to make this the touchstone of the hospital plan. Even more important is the fact that while some GPs want to do hospital work the majority do not, and prefer to be thought of as specialists in domiciliary care rather than as part GPs, part hospital doctor.

The ideal solution is, of course, to have no separation between the GP and the hospital consultant team, to have them working together so closely that they can decide what is best suited to their particular circumstances. There are many new and experimental ideas to be tried and many activities in which the group of general practitioners at one health centre must join. Day hospitals are proving increasingly useful and day surgery, in which minor cases are operated on and returned home the same day to the care of their GPs and the district nurse, who is also supplied with sterile dressings and instruments by the hospital, will surely spread round the country. Night hospitals for those who can still work even while they need some skilled attention are not yet very common in Britain. Then there is the possible development of nursing units in which the doctor plays a very small part; having done what needed his skill urgently, he leaves the rest to qualified nurses at home or in a special unit. The combinations of methods and the variety of possible schemes is almost endless, and awaits only our integration of the services and the establishment of the medical team on the same basis as the nurses and ancillary workers, salaried and full-time.

The Department of Health must in an integrated service go on playing a major role in whatever changes are made in the use of hospitals, and has in the past made it quite clear that it accepts that the development of the district general hospital will mean the closure of some small hospitals. Indeed in 1968 38 hospitals, of which 30 had fewer than 50 beds each, were closed. The Department has stated that before any closure takes place not only must the public know about the proposal but consultations must take place with the local authorities and the general practitioners in the hospital area. Above all the Department has said alternative uses for any hospital which no longer seems essential must be considered. In many areas such hospitals could very well become health centres without much new capital having to be found. The Department is also aware of the need to consider the case for retaining an otherwise not very efficient unit because its disappearance would mean that people had to go to another locality for services and would be involved in transport difficulties and expense. When such matters as these have been considered by the regional hospital board the Secretary of State still has to make the final decision.

The Department of Health would find all this much easier in an integrated service, for the bodies that now have to be consulted would have been replaced, for health purposes, by one organization. It would at that stage be more important than ever that the public should be informed and consulted; and if the district health committee is an elected body this would be the normal procedure and no exhortations would be needed from the centre. The centre, however, must remain responsible for the task of planning the hospitals of the future on new lines, and much research and some experimentation has been done to try to establish what the best design for today is that will not be too out of date at the end of the century when these hospitals will still be the main structures of the hospital service. The Department says that 'increasing emphasis has been placed on standardization and industrialization'. The designers have the difficult task of 'producing standard departmental designs to cover almost all departments of a district general hospital', but progress is being made. That industrialization may be applied to hospital buildings as well as equipment offers the possibility of more flexible and less permanent buildings, or at least greater flexibility within buildings. The hospital service is still trying to do its work in hundreds of old buildings designed for other purposes, which therefore cannot be continually redesigned as the work of a department changes and as new equipment comes forward. The present writer took charge of remodelling old poor-house single-storey wards just after World War II to make a laboratory for a whole group of hospitals. It was inadequate and unsuitable but it was the best available. Twenty years later it is more than inadequate and many times less suitable but it will not be replaced by modern buildings for some eight to ten years yet. In whatever new hospitals are built it is clearly desirable to have some kind of flexibility which will avoid or minimize this kind of thing at the end of this century.

There are, of course, areas in Britain where small hospitals must be retained, for geography makes any other system difficult. But even there the welfare of the patient must be the guide as to what kind of work is to be done in them and by whom. It was the medical profession in Britain which felt that we must get away from the era when general practitioners did their own surgery and we must not allow any suggestion that we slip back to this old position. Specialization has gone too far for that to happen; specialists not only like but need modern equipment, laboratory, X-ray and electronic resources around them, and these must be concentrated where they can be used efficiently and safely. The public will go along with all these ideas if it is told about them and if the medical profession gives a clear lead as to what is best.

Nevertheless we should return to the question of the optimum size of a hospital, for planning will clearly be influenced by any guide that can be given. Opinion since the NHS started has frequently changed but chiefly because no definition has been given as to what we need to provide a comprehensive service. Unless there is much more examination of hospital records and experiments it will be difficult to reach conclusions. The size of wards, the number of single-bed rooms, the amount of recreational space, the way in which sterile supplies are handled and stored, the amount of visiting that is to be permitted, allowing mothers to stay with their children—all affect the size and planning of hospitals. Above all the optimum size for modern laboratories must be taken into account. No hospital can do a comprehensive job today without a complete team of clinical laboratory specialists; but equally no small hospital can possibly demand and use all the resources and techniques a good clinical laboratory can put at the service of a large team of experts in a variety of disciplines.

In speaking of taking the service to the patient or the patient to the service we must not overlook the need for mobile units even in an urban health service, and the need for a very flexible transport and ambulance service. We have more than once suggested that in any country, but particularly in Britain and other western European countries, town and country must be planned for as a unit and this is very important when speaking of the smaller hospital. In so far as they remain and have a variety of purposes their link with the larger units and the more highly specialized ones that deal with emergencies, with trauma, with burns, with the intensive care of heart disease cases and so on must be continuous and rapid. The longer distances in Britain, for instance between the Hebridean Islands and Glasgow, are few and already make use of the aeroplane. There is a strong case for the use of the helicopter to assist with accidents in our mountains and round the coast; for the rest it is essential to have a large enough and fast enough ambulance service. But transport of patients and their relatives must be a freely available service if we are to link our district general hospitals with smaller hospitals and other facilities. Our ambulance personnel are being better trained today than ever before but the experience already gained with mobile units dealing with heart emergencies, and the much wider experience of other countries, notably the USSR, indicate that we should have more nurses and doctors trained and available for mobile and emergency services.

The Department of Health is probably still thinking too much in terms of buildings rather than services; but everyone welcomes decisions made in 1972 to increase further the building programme which had been started by the previous government. The amount spent on buildings was steadily increasing, £85 million in 1967–8 in England, £92 million in 1968–9, and almost exactly £100 million in 1969–70. But more important was that in these years new schemes were initiated and at the end of 1969 £320 million of new building had already been started. The amount which regional hospital boards were spending on schemes not controlled from the centre had also risen. Still the rate was not fast enough and in February 1972 Sir Keith Joseph announced that in the next five years much more, at comparable prices, would be put into the capital programme, partly to meet the increase already in the pipeline because of schemes already started, and partly new spending, making an average annual increase of £50 million, some £800 million in all for the five years. This, with what has been done, will transform many of Britain's oldest hospitals into modern buildings and, if the staffing and maintenance follows, will provide an unequalled service.

Within these hospitals the key figures must be the consultants in charge of beds, and there is no longer any reason why the building and staffing of them should be complicated by trying to retain a small number of private pay beds for the personal enrichment of a few privileged doctors. Without this enormous outpouring of public money on the laboratories, X-ray plants, operating theatres and so on none of the private work could be done, or would earn so much, in such modern buildings. One feature that has been noted is that the wealthy do not turn away from the NHS for many ordinary illnesses and they certainly do not do so in the case of chronic disease, which is not usually covered by their insurance policies. A short, sharp surgical condition which can be paid for by the insurance, the premiums for which were paid by one's employer, is one thing: a long illness or one requiring continuing checks and blood tests, for example, is something the wealthiest know the NHS does better and more cheaply. There is of course a strong public current against private practice because it is synonymous with something the British do not like, queue-jumping. In *Medical World* of March 1972, Dr Hugh Faulkner, Medical Secretary of the Medical Practitioners' Union, wrote: 'There can be no doubt that the majority of citizens disapprove of buying a privileged place in the queue for medical care, and it is deeply resented by many working in the service'.

But a new problem is likely to arise if Britain is part of the Common Market, in defining who is a specialist and who, therefore, should have access to all this subsidy. Since the NHS started a specialist in Britain has been, simply, a man or woman appointed to a specialist post within the NHS. The lines of qualification, training and experience, the higher qualification such as membership or fellowship of a Royal College, have all been well understood by the profession and by the committees appointed by regional boards to make such appointments. There can be no question that the criteria laid down make Britain's consultants among the best trained and qualified men in any hospital service. But the Common Market requires some degree, indeed an almost complete system, of standardized definition of a specialist throughout all the nations concerned. To require that the recognition of specialist rank involves giving full-time service to the NHS, as the majority already do, would make the inevitable negotiations on this matter very much simpler and would give a lead to Europe. The need for sharp definitions is most pressing in those countries where insurance funds pay specialists in accordance with a list of fees different from that applicable to non-specialists. Britain, having a service free of charges and free of private practice, would be ethically and legally in a superior position to all other nations concerned.

Within any hospital system there arise many problems which the medical profession has tried to meet by increasing specialization, but this has not been followed by similar, or at least adequate, developments in buildings and services. We have hinted at the need for day hospitals and night hospitals, and we already have units which are trying to give service to the elderly in new ways. The geriatrician is one of the most recent of specialists, and many other specialists still resist the term because every doctor has to treat elderly people. Still there are problems arising from old age which need social solutions, and while everyone agrees that ideally the elderly must be kept within their own families and their own communities – in which local day hospitals with recreational and rehabilitative services must play a part – there comes the moment when hospitalization of some kind is the only answer. A great deal of new thought, and, as the elderly grow in numbers, a great deal of new money needs to be put into this provision. It must be coupled with similar new ideas to deal with those who are disabled, no matter what the cause of the disablement, or its type, may be. This is one field in which relations must be invited and encouraged to give voluntary assistance within State institutions.

These problems raise one other point about the specialist, and an additional reason why he should be a full-time officer giving equal quality of care to all his patients: the need to develop further the domiciliary consultative service. Nothing separates the British system from the thinking still prevalent in many countries, especially the USA, as much as the idea that consultants should leave their ivory towers and join their GP colleagues in the homes of the sick. This is team-work epitomized and must be developed to the point where it is so much a national procedure that we keep more and more cases at home instead of in a hospital bed, which is much more expensive. Experience in those areas where it has been most highly developed shows that there are many cases, including acute coronary disease, where with proper specialist assessment and consultation it is not only economically and psychologically worth while but clinically much better to keep the patient at home. For some years the number of domiciliary consultations has been around 320,000 and in an integrated service this figure should rise. Indeed it is sometimes objected that the present rate is under twenty per GP each year and that not all are consultations in the true sense because consultant and GP do not meet at the patient's bed. But a high proportion of domiciliary visits are by clinical pathologists and radiologists who cannot 'consult' until they have got the results of their tests after returning to base. More critical is the suggestion that in some areas visits are a device of GPs to get round waiting lists and especially to get elderly patients into hospital. But some of these consultations rightly result in urgent admissions. On the other hand some simply provide help in cases which the GP has already decided can stay at home, and a large proportion result in cases not being admitted, thus saving hospital beds.

Two additional points must be made. Where full postgraduate education is going on at a district general hospital team-work is greatly increased and the GP can be in regular contact with his hospital colleagues. Where small hospitals have been retained and GPs have regular duties there, they will be in very close contact with consultants whether called specially or making regular visits, and much discussion of cases will take place there. It is for these reasons that it is doubtful whether those 'GP hospitals' which exist, and those suggested by some writers, which have no consultant in charge, can be justified if a high standard of care is being attempted.

As well as the domiciliary consultations we must look at the opposite side of the hospital story: waiting lists which are usually around half a million, of which nearly 400,000 are for surgery; and in any year 70,000 waiting for the removal of tonsils and adenoids. This is not a subject for either horror or complacency. It must be recognized that it may not be shortage of beds which produces waiting time, for the daily average of empty surgical beds is over 12,000. There is a large organizational element. There were, in 1969, 1,902,507 discharges and deaths from surgical beds, each of which treated nearly thirty people in the year. There are sometimes serious errors and mistakes in handling waiting lists, but it must be remembered it is the doctor who puts a patient on the waiting list who will have to deal with the case eventually. He is contending daily with urgent and emergency cases and the waiting list, correctly used (and often the name is a misnomer), is a device for smoothing out the work. Sometimes, too, a surgeon may hold up cases, for example tonsils, because there is no point in doing some non-urgent operations at bad, foggy or cold times of the year. Nor does the waiting list stand still: the half-million on the list one day are a different half-million from a week, a month ago.

But it should nevertheless be public policy that there are always beds waiting for patients, not patients waiting for beds. There may at any moment be between 50,000 and 70,000 beds available and not occupied but many are beds in the wrong place for the cases needing them. This is one reason why an emergency bed bureau should be set up in every district, with collaboration between districts, so that beds can be used to the greatest advantage. With greater co-operation between medical teams much can be done; and when there is no private practice within the service there will be no suspicion that waiting lists, and waiting time, are used as reasons for persuading patients to pay a consultant's fee to get a bed without waiting, even for a far from urgent case.

When full-time service becomes the rule the method of payment of specialists, and indeed the whole promotional system, will have to be re-examined. All specialists are eligible for a bonus payment or merit award of which there are four grades, the A plus at the top being equivalent to doubling the full-time salary. These awards are given by a specially appointed medical committee but are not made known to the public. It is probably the only case in which public money is given in secret by a method which has never been revealed.

Each consultant is invited to fill up a form about himself and it is said many resent this and do not do so. Other evidence as to 'merit' is then sought from colleagues and through inquiries made by members of the committee. It inevitably produces many queries, doubts and problems, especially as men working together in a hospital team cannot know who has got a reward or of what size—most are of the lowest grade C. It is possible for a relatively junior man in a department to have a reward about which his senior colleague, who does not have a reward, knows nothing. The published list of awards according to specialty shows that the distribution is not even as to region, as to age of first award, or as to type of specialty. Thus only 12.2 per cent of geriatricians have an award as against 70.0 per cent of cardiologists; 18.8. per cent of anaesthetists against 78.6 per cent of thoracic surgeons; 21.1 per cent of specialists in mental health but 63.4 per cent of neurologists. These anomalies are incidental to a system which can have no place in an integrated service in which team-work, not rivalry, is the keynote. The money should be used to produce a better overall system of payment, a good promotional ladder, and such additional payments as should attach to particular posts, either for extra skill and experience or because administration, research or advisory work is undertaken.

Behind these discussions one must visualize the millions of citizens who have had on average one hospital out-patient attendance each year and one admission to a hospital bed each eight years or so (the lucky ones having very much less, the unlucky ones not only having more admissions but a much longer time in hospital care). It is for them that the hospitals of AD 2,000 have to be planned, but have to be planned now. We must assume that national wealth goes on increasing, is better distributed and better spent: we cannot conclude that hospitals will be required any less than today. Some diseases may disappear, although surprisingly a recent estimate shows at least 100 new cases of tuberculosis being diagnosed in AD 2,000 in Britain. So hospitals, which must be functional, must also be designed to make those visits, which to the patient are so important, as free from troubles as we can make them. Every detail needs to be checked by people who can project themselves into the position of the sick, the lame, the blind, the shy and the frightened. These are the things most people bring up when they complain about hospitals being too big, too cold, too inhuman. Design plus people trained to serve must carry the NHS hospitals into a future for which new superlatives will have to be found.

Chapter 12

Out-of-Hospital Care

We have given this chapter a title intended to link with Chapter 11, but it does not really describe what remains to be discussed. It seems to imply that the hospital provides the dividing line between two types of service, but this is not really so, for the patient who needs both in-hospital and out-of-hospital care is one and the same. As René Dubos has put it in *Man, Medicine, and Environment* (1968), 'whatever the complaints of the patient and the signs or symptons he manifests, whatever the medical problems of the community, disease cannot be understood or successfully controlled without considering man in his total environment'. It is true that this view 'corresponds to an abstract ideal not amenable to full achievement in practice either by the clinician or the public health officer'. The writer goes on to suggest that many of the problems cannot yet be fully understood and the environment cannot be fully controlled, and always, whatever the technological position, 'the art of medicine consists to a large extent in the ability of medical men to devise practical measures best suited to the human beings involved'. It is that fact, that we are dealing with human beings, which has never to be forgotten in planning services and it becomes increasingly difficult when we reach our present-day position in which one doctor can no longer attempt to deal with all the modern complexities. Away from the philosophical attitudes which René Dubos discusses, 'what is obvious is that the days of the single-handed physician or the over-restricted group are over', as John Fry says in *Medicine in Three Societies* (1969). He goes on: 'Work in this field [outside the hospital] requires a team of physicians, nurses, social workers and others, just as much as does the work in hospitals.' There is still a dilemma for the individual doctor wherever he works but especially when his work is in the heart of his community in a continuing relationship, as opposed to the episodic position of the hospital specialist. As Max Rosenheim has put it (*WHO Chronicle*, February 1961), 'The doctor of the future must be leader of a team'. We are now 'entering an era in which total medical and social care is likely to be provided by team-work but the practising doctor must remain the friend and personal adviser of the individual patient'.

It was for these and other reasons discussed earlier that the British NHS was firmly founded on the general practitioners. They were, at that time, the largest voice in medicine, and among the senior doctors of the country still are, even if the NHS has doubled the number of consultants, and there was a strong bias in their favour. Everything written in the five years before the NHS was written as if no other system could be contemplated. The BMA's Medical Planning Commission (1942) certainly voiced the general feeling when it said:

> There seems to be general agreement that the organization of the national health services should be based upon the family as the normal unit and on the family doctor as the normal medical attendant and guardian. The first essential is not institutional but personal service, such as can be rendered by a family doctor who has the continuous care of the health of the family under his charge.

When we come to write of the future we may need to elaborate on the widening range of duties of the future family doctor, but few would quarrel with the BMA's 1942 definition: 'The GP will afford them [his patients] such professional services as he can render personally and will make it his duty to see that they obtain full advantage of all the further auxiliary services that may be otherwise provided.' To some members of the Medical Planning Commission, as its *Draft Interim Report* records, it seemed that all that and 'team work, correlation and co-ordination, easier opportunities of regular postgraduate study, pension schemes and freedom from financial worry' could best be achieved by a salaried service, but the majority thought otherwise.

It is still a subject for final settlement. In health centres, which we discuss in this chapter, a salaried service would be ideal and would obviate many difficulties, remove rivalry and get rid of the question of private practice which is incompatible with the team spirit in a health centre employing many salaried health workers. (Private practice has, as Irvine and Jefferys have recorded (*British Medical Journal*, 1971, 4, 535), 'declined dramatically. In 1963, 77 per cent had private patients, 14 per cent more than 100. In 1968 only 58 per cent had any and only 5 per cent more than 100'.) Since the NHS started general practitioners have been paid by an increasingly complicated method but have in effect received regular payments and have a final annual settlement of details. The GP gets money from the State for at least thirty different reasons, including such small sums spread over all England and Wales as £1,032 for helping dentists to arrest dental haemorrhage and £6,457 for giving anaesthetics. However over £80 million, out of £107 million, is paid for basic practice allowances, for ordinary capitation fees and temporary residents and maternity services. There is another £10 million for seniority and supplementary fees which could easily be adjusted for in any salaried service. The GPs asked for this system, without perhaps appreciating its complexities, in order to ensure 'clinical freedom' which, it was imagined, would not be possible in a salaried service. Since then the hospital service has demonstrated that complete clinical freedom is not only possible but enhanced by a salaried service; and even a bonus scheme, if GPs wanted such a thing, is possible.

It was for all these reasons that health centres were to be established. The Medical Planning Commission had come out heavily in favour of health centres, which 'must on the one hand preserve the professional independence of the co-operating general practitioners and must on the other hand be capable of becoming an organized unit in an integrated medical service'. The desire of the majority of the Commission was to emphasize 'co-operation' rather than the public provision, which the minority demanded, of 'a health unit in which health centres would be linked with the hospitals, assume the duties of certain special clinics, co-operate in matters of public health and ensure for all a complete domiciliary consultant and institutional service'. That was in fact almost a plea for the integrated service that has been under discussion ever since; and when the Labour Government introduced the NHS it was that minority view, pressed on the Commission by known Labour Party members, which became the law. But that law has never been realized and even in 1972 is not understood by many, irrespective of their view of health centres: so it is as good a place as any to start looking at the future of health care.

There is a difference between the Health Service Acts for England and Wales and for Scotland: in the latter health centres are provided by the central authority, in England and Wales by the local health authority, usually the county council. The Scottish system has resulted in better planning and more complete realization of what was intended in the clauses of the original Acts. We need not repeat the parliamentary phraseology but Clause 21 of the 1946 Act gives a complete description of what was to be the clear duty of the health authority in England and Wales: 'to provide, equip and maintain' buildings for general services, medical, dental, pharmaceutical, local authority services and for the service of specialists or anyone else provided by the hospitals. Even more important, for all the above go together, was section (f), 'for the publication of information on questions relating to health or disease, and for the delivery of lectures and the display of pictures or cinematograph films in which such questions are dealt with'. And to attend to all this the local authority had the duty to provide any staff necessary (except those provided by hospitals or the local executive council services).

We need not now go into all the political, social and economic reasons why these provisions were not carried out at once. Preliminary plans of buildings, the marking out of sites and calculations as to numbers of people to be served were all put on paper and then put in pigeon-holes somewhere until the continuous propaganda for health centres, which never ceased, plus the movement of opinion inside the medical profession, caused new plans to be produced. The Medical Planning Commission had hinted that 'in some areas practitioners may wish to anticipate a statutory scheme and establish health centres by voluntary co-operation'. The profession itself accepted that, except in rural areas, the single-handed practice was no longer right, and rapidly moved into forms of group practice, sometimes acquiring premises that might be classified as health centres except that they did not carry the other services which the Act envisaged. By 1971 not more than 16 per cent of all family doctors were in single-handed practice; and the NHS made money available to enable alterations to be made to practice premises.

In the first eighteen years of the NHS only thirty-three health centres were opened but from 1965 onwards encouragement was given to local authorities to go ahead, and the profession demanded progress, and by the end of 1971 there were over 280 health centres open in England and Wales. Even more important was the fact that over 200 more were already being built or were about to be built. Lord Aberdare, Minister of State in the Department of Health, was able to say in February 1972: 'There is continuing and strong demand and my Department has information which suggests that the demand is in fact increasing every year.' He anticipated that by the end of 1974 there would be over 500 health centres functioning, but this rate of development will probably be too slow as public and professions learn in practice the advantages of health centre services. Demand will certainly grow for the more rapid development of the other services; dental care in health centres would be an enormous boon to the whole population, and in many areas not only the pharmacist but other services could be included. Lord

Aberdare appeared to have accepted the concept of health centres in its entirety, for he went on to say that he was anxious to maintain the impetus that had been given to building because 'when we can bring together family doctors, other community health workers and, where appropriate, social work staff in a single purpose-built building, and when these dedicated people work together as a community team, I believe that we make a very real contribution to the health of the community'.

We are however for the moment concerned rather with the disease diagnosis and treatment services, and there can be no question in anyone's mind that the doctor's way of life is enormously improved by health centre practice and that he can give better service to his patients by having in the same building help from many ancillary health workers. Much of that help will have to be worked out in practice and there will undoubtedly be much variation and some experimentation. The family doctor's role, which we will discuss later, will change, but so will the role and work of the health visitor, the nurse and the midwife. They too have often been isolated and single-handed and the correct relationship between themselves and the general practitioners has had to be established on an individual basis. Much thought will have to be given to the role of those ancillary staff who share the general practitioner's domiciliary work. This must remain, and indeed develop, as the most important part of their joint efforts. They, rather than any academic work study group, must work out what the nurse can do to relieve the doctor, especially if there is, as so frequently happens in winter in Britain, a large increase in infections. It is now accepted that from training and experience many nurses can make a tentative diagnosis, institute immediate treatment and report to the doctor, as she can now do so easily at the health centre. There would appear to be no place in Britain for the type of paramedical worker now being trained in America (and who is undoubtedly useful in the underdeveloped countries with few doctors), to replace the GPs as the primary care worker, to do the home visiting. With her own group of doctors the well-trained nurse can do all and much more than 'sub-physicians' acting quite independently because she will be doing her work as a member of an integrated team. That team in future must also include some of the hospital nurses, especially those with experience in the nursing of children and in midwifery, to come out into the community when necessary and back up the domiciliary team.

There is a danger in continually referring to community care that some people may elevate it to another form of specialization. What the future needs is that every health worker is fully aware of his or her relation to the community, of the importance of community care and the paramount need to build up a healthy community in which all citizens are given whatever care they need. It may be seen that it would be an error to cease having within every community a Medical Officer of Health whose only patient was the community as a whole, for someone must look at the health of a whole human unit just as the doctor responsible for any form of treatment must look at the patient as a whole. The family doctor must be the physician of primary contact but he is best suited, and in a health centre, best provided with assistance to be the true community physician. Nevertheless the team may need someone quite free from the problems of sick individuals because community problems become more and more complex. Greenholm and Draper have said that 'there is a pressing requirement in health care systems to cope with the variability and uniqueness that characterize the consumer, whether the recipient is an individual patient, a neighbourhood or a region'. The family doctor will see the problem from within, as it were, and the more he is aware of being a community physician the better. But someone else with knowledge of mass problems may also have to stand a little aside and look into the community so that he can identify the matters that need his special form of care.

All of this will become much clearer and simpler when we have an integrated service, and many problems as to duties and work will disappear once all the staff of the health service, employed by the service, are paid on the same full-time basis—that is, the whole of the time they spend on health care (whether part- or full-time) is given to the service, without any private practice or other health care source of income. Salary and promotional scales, which we have yet to discuss, will also become simpler. Perhaps some of the other troubles that arise in our general health care services would disappear. The general practitioner has been much criticized and the centre of many arguments over the prescription of drugs. The prescription of medicines is of course vital to a primary care physician, and in Britain he has had the liberty to prescribe at the expense of a third party (national health insurance or NHS) for his patients since 1911. His prescriptions cost many millions of pounds every year more than he himself earns. He writes about 250 million prescriptions a year and out of that nearly 175 million will be for proprietary preparations costing on average up to five times what non-proprietary drugs cost. He writes only 5.27 prescriptions a year per patient in the West Midlands but 6.10 in the North-West. He writes 69 million prescriptions for drugs acting on the nervous system but only half that number for infections and only about 19 million for heart and related diseases. He is free to do all this but his figures are checked and theoretically he should not exceed the average number for his own area. In 1969, for example, 1,135 doctors had figures higher than the average and a regional medical officer called on every one to ask him why. That the faults were not too serious must be assumed as only six cases were referred to the adjudicating local medical committee (for this is done by the medical profession, not the Government), and three doctors were fined by the Secretary of State through the withholding of part of their salary (two between £10 and £25, but one as much as £600).

There are other causes for investigation by local executive councils of the work of GPs, and these arise from a variety of allegations as to a breach of contract. It must be remembered that the GP works under a contract of service, and in any year between 500 and 600 breaches of contract may be investigated for doctors, between 200 and 300 for dentists, and small numbers for opticians and pharmacists. Most years in some three-quarters of cases no breach of contract is proved; and the others range from cases in which a fine of under £100 by withholding income is the result, to a very few in which stronger action, even cancellation of the contract, is taken. The medical profession has not yet realized that the policing of its own members which it has done since 1911 arises from reasons and causes that have no place in the salaried hospital service and would have no place if their anachronistic contract of service was replaced by national employment. Doctors in the hospital service also prescribe drugs but they have available the information and pharmacist advice that enables them to watch out for errors and abuses.

It should be noted that two items which increase the health service bureaucracy in unnecessary ways are the Dental Estimates Board and the Pricing Bureaux which have the task of pricing prescriptions and paying the retail pharmacists. When there is a universal system of health centres and all have their pharmacist this will be greatly diminished or will disappear. The Dental Estimates Board has a staff of over 1,200 to deal with the approval of those items of care that require prior approval and to price the cost of dental care, approximately £75 million, including the increasing amount, around £20 million, paid by the patients. Dentistry is a very important item in health care and one which by its very nature, its variability, the need for prophylaxis, the number of painful emergencies, the appliances that can now be supplied and so on, is pre-eminently suited to a free-of-charges system. The fee per item of service, with or without a charge paid by the patient, is complicated, difficult and expensive to operate and leads to many appeals by dentists against decisions made by the Dental Estimates Board. For example in 1969 there were 650 appeals, of which approximately 180 were decided in favour of the appellant, 220 in favour of the Board, 70 or so partly in favour of each, with the rest still outstanding at the end of the year. In a salaried service there might need to be some safeguards but the dentist would be expected to have the same integrity as, say, the surgeon in hospital, to do all that was necessary but to avoid unnecessary procedures and at all times to avoid pain and trauma which could be avoided. One fault in the dental service today is that the method of payment and the need for estimates have led many dentists either to say they carry out certain procedures only on a private fee basis or to persuade patients to be treated as wholly private cases. Full-time dentistry in well-equipped health centres is beyond question the only answer.

The dentist should, of course, also be part of that team which is looking after the health of a community. Dental care, especially in children, is a vital part of health care, and in an integrated service new arrangements will have to be made to combine school dental services, general dental care and orthodontic work so that children get really complete attention at all times. Every country in the world would appear to be short of fully qualified dentists. In the US it is part of the proposals for universally available service that only priority classes, in the first instance children up to twelve years, will get full dental care under the insurance scheme. In Britain we have begun to make good use of the dental hygienist but we need more of them and of dental technicians as well as qualified dentists.

In the final analysis so much of community health is environmental and may be damaged by an imperfect or polluted neighbourhood. All health workers have to be alerted to faults that may make health less certain or life more hazardous. Education of health workers in all the hazards of modern industrialization is therefore important and must be so orientated as to lead to an advance in that social responsibility and co-operation with the people which is essential to improvements in individual and community health.

Chapter 13

The Supporting Services

The British NHS is rightly spoken of as one of our largest industries and some of the figures in the many tables in the annual report of the Department of Health and Social Security give some idea of how wide ranging an industry it is, in terms both of manpower and of materials. The ambulances, both those for emergencies and for non-urgent transport, travelled over 129 million miles and carried well over 21 million cases in a year. The National Blood Transfusion Service collected over one and a half million bottles of blood and distributed most of it in a fresh state, but also some as plasma and other products to hospitals all over the country. The laboratories dealt with more than 37 million individual requests for tests and used a lot of equipment, for example, they made a contract for nearly £3 million for equipment and £2.5 million for disposable syringes and needles between laboratories and hospitals. X-ray departments had over 31 million patients and ordered £6 million of X-ray film and paper and over £4 million of new equipment. The physiotherapy departments had, between groups and individuals, over 13 million attendances and, sad but remarkable, 19,000 artificial legs and arms were provided. To keep all that going and quite apart from the professional and technical staff, about 35,000 of them, there were 61 other grades of employees, works, maintenance and domestic totalling over 190,000 full-time equivalents. (There are high numbers of part-time workers especially on the domestic side.)

It is not always appreciated that behind the surgeon about to operate there are a whole host of people directly and indirectly making the operation and its success possible. Conversely, however, there are in the whole service only two people employed for each hospital bed. It is a paradoxical service which may need twenty or more people to manage one episode in the life of one person, yet manages its millions of treatments, tests and X-rays and covers the health of the children at school and the families at home with an average of one person employed for every fifty potential patients.

The doctor, not only as leader of the modern team but as the most highly trained, and highest paid, of all these workers, is in the final analysis the man for whom all these supporting services have to be supplied. But we must not overlook that some of the other health workers, the dentists, the opticians, many health visitors and district nurses, also undertake quite independent forms of health care; and though they may refer cases to doctors or ask for medical assistance with some problems, they are not working under medical supervision. There is in every part of the health service a subtle and largely unwritten division of labour and responsibility, much of which has developed over many years and is understood by members of the team even if it would be difficult to put into precise terms. Relationships of this nature are much more easily developed in a service when all are working under the same financial arrangements and the question of charges, private or public, therefore does not interfere with the professional relationship.

So it is accepted that the modern doctor needs all these supporting services. In the hospitals of the country most are fully developed in the district general hospitals, teaching hospitals and other large institutions but have to be organized for smaller places. Today the consultants in the hospital service take it for granted that X-ray departments and all kinds of laboratories are available to do any of the multiplicity of tests that may be demanded. Neither is a very old development, both grew slowly in the first thirty years of the century, both have seen tremendous growth rates in the last forty years. There were some services in the larger voluntary hospitals but very little among the poor-law hospitals until they were municipalized in 1929. They had hardly begun to develop laboratories and it was out of this scarcity that the author in that year suggested the problem would best be solved by group laboratories, each serving a number of hospitals. The London County Council, which had taken over some seventy-five hospitals, began with five group laboratories and a large central laboratory for diagnostic histology, which could be centralized more easily than much of the clinical laboratory work. The group laboratory concept began to spread all over the country and was given great impetus when the Emergency Hospital Service was set up to prepare for World War II. When in 1948 the NHS began to organize its hospital groups, each to be controlled by a hospital group management committee, the laboratory service already had in many areas the pattern that suited and which is now the rule.

One of the important developments between 1935 and the introduction of the NHS was the increasing use of laboratories by the general practitioners. In voluntary hospitals the honorary pathologist usually made the whole or part of his living from fees collected from public health authorities who needed his aid with infectious diseases, diphtheria, tuberculosis and so on, and from fees paid by the private patients of the other hospital consultants. But the hitherto untapped source of work from family doctors was developed by an offer from pathologists of what came to be known as 'an open access service' in which whatever work was needed was done for such fees as the GP thought could be charged or no fee in poorer cases. Once again wartime stimulated this and as most pathologists had been enrolled in the Emergency Hospital Service and were being paid as if in the army, the charging of fees became of minor importance; and by the end of the war county councils were offering full-time employment to those who had manned the laboratories which had become associated with the larger former poor-law institutions rather than the smaller voluntary hospitals.

Today the whole of Britain is covered by a double chain of laboratories, for World War II produced the necessity for and saw the growth of the Public Health Laboratory Service. It began because some bacteriologists recognized, and persuaded the Government to recognize, that if the war produced epidemics of infectious disease, or if water and food became infected, special laboratories equipped for the identification of bacteria, and later, viruses, would be needed. Technically this is not a part of the NHS but it is so closely used by the laboratories of the NHS for reference purposes in bacterial and viral diseases that it is only in its administration, control and finance that it is separate. Indeed many of the laboratories of the PHLS are at or form part of hospital laboratories with interlocking staff and duties. It may be added that the laboratories of the PHLS are the seat of a large part of Britain's research in all matters relating to infectious diseases. It provides a very good example of a health service which can only be organized on a national basis, and is almost unique in its potential for dealing with such epidemics as we still get.

The hospital laboratories have increased in staff, size of buildings, capital value of equipment and in every other way. The staff of consultant pathologists has more than doubled since the NHS began, but much more spectacular has been the increase in the number of technicians and scientific officers which the laboratories now employ. The rising costs of all hospital care are also reflected in rising laboratory costs but in some ways they are surprisingly low. In 1970–1 the element in the cost of an in-patient per week in an acute hospital was £2.34 which would appear to be not too high for a very fine standard of scientific work. The unit used in assessing costs is 100 'weighted' requests which on average was £16.62, and the cost per case was £3.54. Many tests are individually costly but there is an increasing use of automatic machines coupled with computers which enable large numbers of the same test to be done at one time.

In any discussion on the place of either X-ray or laboratory in the work of the physician of primary contact, the important question is whether he has open access in the double sense that he can get done those things he considers will be of diagnostic assistance (and here the absence of fees is of enormous importance compared with countries where such tests have to be paid for), and also that he can consult the laboratory workers over what should be done and how results should be interpreted. Pathologists in Britain have always insisted that theirs is in a clinical discipline and if this is to be so the relationship between laboratory workers and all doctors, but above all the family doctors, must be close. Quite a high proportion of domiciliary consultations are done by clinical pathologists, both for diagnostic purposes and for control of the type of treatment, for diabetes, for anti-coagulant therapy in cardio-vascular disease and so on. The amount of use made by family doctors varies widely but at present the national average is that about 12 per cent of the laboratory services' individual requests are for general practitioners.

The pattern for X-ray examinations is surprisingly similar, the proportion of work referred directly by GPs being a little higher than for pathology; and the amount of emergency work, especially if there is a large accident and casualty department in a hospital, is higher than in the laboratory. One of the problems arising from the need to have both these services on a twenty-four-hour basis is that of staffing. The laboratory technician and the radiographer both have to be on emergency call or actually on duty to cover a larger part of the day than would ordinary 'office hours'; and consultants in both disciplines have to man emergency services since urgent expert advice has become a true necessity of both medicine and surgery.

Part of the supporting service that is vital but purely hospital in scope, is blood transfusion. The National Blood Transfusion Service is now over forty years old. The first big test of blood transfusion under modern warfare conditions was in the Spanish Civil War from which British doctors brought back a warning, and experience of what might be expected. Today no one questions the outstanding quality of blood transfusion work in the UK, or fails to recognize how well it is organized. In his study of the subject, *The Gift Relationship* (1971), Professor R. M. Titmuss found that social policy closely affects both the quantity and the quality of blood obtained. He compared the unpaid donor system of Britain with the system of buying and selling blood in America and concluded that amongst other things

> the commercialization of blood and donor relationships represses the expansion of altruism, erodes the sense of community, lowers scientific standards, limits both personal and professional freedoms, sanctions the making of profits in hospitals and clinical laboratories, legalizes hostility between doctor and patient, subjects critical areas of medicine to the laws of the market-place, places immense social costs on those least able to bear them – the poor, the sick and the inept – increases the danger of unethical behaviour in various sectors of medical science and practice. . . .

No such criticism can be directed against the National Blood Transfusion Service which is entirely dependent on volunteer donors and has a scientific reputation unexcelled. It is organized regionally for collection and storage purposes and each of the regional depots is responsible for ensuring supplies to the laboratories in each hospital group. The responsibility for cross-matching the blood for individual patients, an essential part of transfusion, is the responsibility of the hospital laboratories, but the experts at the blood depots are available to advise in difficult cases, to provide blood of very special groups or to overcome any difficulty in cross-matching. It should be mentioned that not only can the various depots in Britain help one another with supplies and rare bloods but there is a close link with the services in Europe and information is exchanged, and if necessary blood. This is a very economically run service and Professor Titmuss found that a commercial system like that in America 'in terms of price per unit of blood to the patient is five to fifteen times more costly than the voluntary system in Britain'. Blood is mainly used in exactly the form in which it is taken from the donor and has a life in the refrigerator of only three weeks. The future may see it preserved for much longer and used in many more varied ways, but from British experience it must remain a voluntary service based on this ethical altruism which is basic to British thinking on the whole subject of medical care.

Blood must be taken with precautions to keep it sterile. The whole question of asepsis, of operating without the danger of infection, the use of antiseptics to destroy germs and the use of antibiotics when an infection does occur has completely altered the atmosphere in a modern hospital compared with even thirty years ago. Surgeons have of course been demanding sterile instruments ever since germs were discovered, but methods were often inefficient and in terms of modern technology used valuable nursing personnel for a task which is more related to the work of the bacteriologist than that of the nurse. So in the last twenty years, accelerating very rapidly over the last ten, the sterilization of instruments and materials has become very much the affair of the laboratory, and of the consultant bacteriologist in particular. As a result most hospitals already have or plan to have a central sterile supply department; and many new techniques for the packaging, sterilizing and delivery of everything the doctor, nurse or technician needs have been developed.

The hospital is, however, not the only place in which sterile instruments and materials are needed, and now the spread of central sterile supplies is seen to be necessary in every field, including that of the general practitioner and the nurse or midwife who goes into the home. Commercial interests as well as hospital sterile supply units now supply many packaged goods, sterilized by gamma radiation, one of the techniques made possible by the use of atomic energy. Most of these sterile packages are enclosed in paper bags and much research has been done by hospital personnel and paper manufacturers to find the ideal paper for this purpose. Most of it is now controlled by British Standard Specifications and the Central Sterilizing Club annually reviews new techniques and materials.

One of the side effects of sterilizing everything in a hospital, or a group of hospitals or, as in the case of Glasgow, a region, has been to produce modifications in hospital design. At one time every ward and unit had to have at least one machine to sterilize instruments by boiling water—not very efficient, a great consumer of heat, very harmful to paintwork, and needing a special room away from the ward. All this has vanished from new hospitals and even from most of Britain's old ones, and in various ways the saving of nurse time and changes in the use of space have produced new possibilities in planning operating theatres, casualty departments and ward units. It also adds a new element to the complex pattern of employees in the health service, groups of workers who work in some ways like production-belt workers in a factory. This is now being developed in many countries but is another field in which British hospitals have a big lead.

It could possibly be argued that many other items in the health service, physiotherapy and now rehabilitation, the provision of appliances, the service of deaf aids and so on are all in a supporting service position but need not be discussed in detail as they are an integral part of the hospital service. New developments, such as the use of computers, may have to be built up as an adjunct both to the laboratories and the clinical services and must affect any future plans for the NHS. That they are powerful possible weapons is unquestioned and already many are in use on the administrative and records side of the service. In building up health records, for the individual and for the nation, the computer is clearly going to make for greater speed and greater action, both necessary in a health service.

Chapter 14

Mental Health

This chapter is really about mental disease, using the term in its widest sense, but no one ever talks about the subject, nor is legislation ever passed about it, except as 'mental health'. There is a great lack of agreement among those who write on the subject as to how much departure from 'normal' there is in the population as a whole; and many estimates are given, for example about how much mental aberration of different kinds the GP will have to deal with in his ordinary practice. John Fry (*Medicine in Three Societies*) estimates that between 10 and 15 per cent of a GP's work will be 'concerned with the management of definite mental illnesses'. We know that almost half the hospital beds in the NHS are for mental cases, the annual admission being of the order of 180,000. The gross expenditure on mental illness and the mentally handicapped is around £140 million each year plus a certain amount for units now part of a general hospital. But the local health authorities are also responsible for the mentally disordered who are in residential care at home and for whom training and education is provided, and these also number about 180,000. The local health authorities have also to provide for many blind, deaf, epileptic and physically handicapped. Then there is the problem of the aged, those whose main symptom of old age is some form of disorientation, and who form a very large proportion both of those in the mental institutions of the hospital service and in the hostels of the local authorities. The NHS also has the responsibility for the special hospitals in which criminals found to be mentally abnormal are detained, over 2,000 at any one time. There is little agreement among experts as to how much real mental disease there is in the country for it is still not accepted as being like physical illnesses, and there is therefore a considerable amount of concealment by patients and their friends and relations. On the other hand society does now recognize a large number of variations in behaviour, including such deviations as homosexuality, as quite separate from mental disease and to be regarded as a social problem rather than as a departure from health.

This changing attitude on the part of society is one of the most dramatic changes since the NHS began. It partly stems from changes which the NHS made possible, and legal enactments like the 1959 Mental Health Act, but it is also part of the general social upheaval we have seen since 1945. The public has in these years become much more tolerant and great efforts have been made to modify the harshness that pervaded institutions for the insane. Parallel with these changes new treatments, particularly with drugs, have greatly reduced the need to isolate the mentally sick from the community, and many experiments in Britain in recent years have shown that large numbers of both the mentally handicapped and the mentally ill can be considered suitably for treatment at home or in their local hospital. The bringing of mental illness into units of the acute general hospitals is increasingly modifying the attitude of patients, the public and even the doctors to the whole subject. The greatest effect of the 1959 Act was undoubtedly that it made it possible for the vast majority of those diagnosed as mentally sick, and needing to be under the control of a psychiatrist, to be admitted to hospital, or in most cases to leave hospital, without formality, and above all without a door being locked behind them. The removal of that fear has in itself helped the mentally sick. The figures for those actually in hospital at the end of 1969, from the annual report of the Department of Health, are given in Table 14.1, and show what

Table 14.1 Legal Status of All Patients in Psychiatric Beds on 31 December 1969

Status	*All categories*	*Mental illness*	*Psychopathic disorder*	*Mental handicap*	*Severe mental handicap*	*Others*
Informal	157,388	98,629	1,110	12,385	44,693	571
Detained under short compulsory powers	1,656	1,608	27	12	3	6
Under other compulsory powers	9,802	5,374	707	1,703	2,007	11
Totals	168,846	105,611	1,844	14,100	46,703	588

a large proportion of all cases were admitted on an informal basis. One can say that very few mental hospitals now present the picture of wards with locked doors, and certainly not for the majority of patients. The public is very conscious of this change and although there are still black spots and have been a few cases of very old-fashioned ideas in very old buildings, on the whole it is accepted that mental disease no longer has the stigma it once bore or causes the fear it once did.

In Britain the ascertainment of mental illness is fairly high whereas in many countries, especially underdeveloped areas with largely rural populations, mental illness is usually hidden unless it takes a violent form. The public attitude to mentally handicapped children has varied greatly in this country but has now definitely swung in favour of retaining in the family and community all who can be sufficiently educated and trained. Who should look after the mentally handicapped is still debated and it is suggested that the education and training of the mentally handicapped should be an educational, not a medical question. In some countries, for example, in the USSR, this makes accurate figures on the mentally handicapped difficult to get for the cases are seen simply as rather bad educational problems. In many countries such mental health services as exist are almost entirely custodial and the care of the mentally sick is still behind locked doors. It is a field in which comparison is almost impossible, for few observers have visited the mental hospitals of foreign countries. Indeed unless one asks specifically to be shown mental hospitals they may not be mentioned. In the erudite study on *The Organization of Medical Care under Social Security* (1969) by Milton I. Roemer, there is no mention of mental health care in any of the eight countries studied. B. Abel-Smith has tried to make a comparison by looking at how much different countries spend on their psychiatric hospitals, and his figures are quoted in Table14.2;

Table 14.2 Cost of Care in Psychiatric Hospitals (1961 or nearest)

Country	*Average cost per bed-day*		*Average cost per bed-day as % of daily per capita national income*
Canada	C$	5.4	128
Czechoslovakia	Kčs	37.1	104
Israel	I£	15.3	298
Philippines	Peso	7.3	619
Poland	Zl	53.1	135
UK	£	1.3	113
USA	$	6.7	103
Yugoslavia	Din.	1,400	293

but before discussing them we should recall that in Britain today much less is spent on mental than on general hospitals. As with all other costs the mental hospital bed costs much more, but its relationship with the cost of a bed in an acute general hospital, 27 per cent only, has not altered. One reason why mental illness and handicapped beds cost so much less it that they have fewer doctors per patient and of course very much less of the supportive services we have already discussed. There are laboratories in new mental service and in places a great deal of investigation, especially biochemical research is being done to try to discover chemical clues to mental sickness; but there is nothing like the same equipment and staff per patient. Discussing the point in *Labour and Inequality* (1972) Nicholas Bosanquet says that although the number of doctors specializing in mental illness has risen, 'it is still worrying that numbers of doctors grew less rapidly than overall'. The blame, he feels, does not all lie with the Government, but 'if doctors by their choice of speciality have voted with their feet against certain types of hospital, it becomes extremely difficult to improve staffing in them'.

It is against that background that we must look at Abel-Smith's figures. The bed-day cost in Britain is more than double the 1961 figure by 1969, but this is true for all hospital figures in all these countries. The relationship is not much altered but unfortunately these costs do not really reflect what one knows about mental health care in the UK and elsewhere.

Any question of comparison is complicated by the fact that the picture of diagnosis and treatment is nowhere so clear or so agreed upon as in purely physical ailments. The field is constantly changing and at the same time the amount of mental illness appears to be on the increase in most modern societies. In spite of this the aim in Britain is definitely to reduce the number of beds in large mental hospitals and replace them with psychiatric units in general hospitals and with care in the community. In physical ailments the aim is always to effect a cure, but in both mental illness and mental deficiency the principal aim is to change the mental state or train the subnormal so that they can live within the community; or if not can at least achieve some kind of life within their own hospital or hostel environment. The use of hostels is of course recognized but, as Elizabeth Durkin puts it in the Fabian Society pamphlet *Hostels for the Mentally Disordered* (1971), 'Hostels are but part of the spectrum of care for the mentally ill'. Hostels have to be backed by other facilities and 'in particular there must be group homes to receive residents from the rehabilitation hostels when they reach a stage at which they can cope with an increase in stress'.

All of this and much more is common ground among those trying to improve the care of the mentally sick and successive Secretaries of State have declared that more money is to be spent in this direction. Thus in November 1971 Sir Keith Joseph announced extra spending over the next four years 'on improving specific health and personal social services, mainly for the elderly and the mentally ill'. His announcement, however, only served to illustrate how much remains to be done, and emphasized how interlinked the care of the aged is with the care of the mentally sick. Much of the increase in spending was earmarked to ensure 'that local authorities will join in a determined effort to sweep away all the former poor-law institutions still being used as old people's homes and replace them with modern buildings'. The Secretary of State rightly described many of the places still being used to accommodate old people, often with severe mental disorientation, as old and unsatisfactory adapted houses which still had Dickensian associations. But many exposures of mental institutions reveal that patients in them still suffer from lack of space, lack of personal possessions which would assist them to be persons, lack of rehabilitation and education. Unless conditions for patients are improved and a great improvement in the training and conditions of employment of staff of all grades is achieved, the increasing number of people who spend a large part of their lives in institutions will always result in a service for which the staff is inadequate. The low spending on psychiatric hospital beds reflects this and much more money than any Secretary of State has provided will need to be available if all the needs are to be met. This shortage of staff often raises the question of how we can reconcile the enormous number of unemployed in the country with underemployment in the service.

This is one field in which there are many groups of citizens who have formed associations to advocate improvements in mental health services and who claim that the answer to the problem is to put people before psychiatry. Since it is asserted that a very high proportion of people will suffer some kind of mental stress and a high proportion of the population will at some point in their lives receive advice and treatment on their mental state, this is a part of the health service in which even more than any other the people must be involved. The involvement usually has to be on a family level: but we now expect it to be on a community level as well. Kenneth Robinson when Minister of Health declared that 'unless community services are provided the community tolerance on which this policy depends will be severely strained'. In the community there will need to be close co-operation and understanding between those giving service in the home, and the family doctor will need to be better equipped to deal with that 10 to 15 per cent of his work said to be of a psychological nature. There are those who would add a great deal of psychological symptoms to that workload and as John Fry has put it, 'the doctor-of-first-contact will have an important role in providing support and care for the less serious disorders that account for most mental illness', *Medicine in Three Societies*. He goes on to emphasize however, that there needs to be much closer co-operation between the specialist psychiatrist and the GP, and this will become possible as more of mental illness is dealt with at district hospitals. In the UK less than 5 per cent of the people the GP considers to have at least psychoneurotic symptoms are sent to see the specialists, and one factor in this we have already mentioned—the relative scarcity of consultants in mental health, approximately 1,000, a little more than one-tenth of all consultants, although they have nearly half the hospital beds in their care. When we consider that they should be as much as possible in the community assisting in early treatment, but above all seeing that the prevention of illness and the education of the sick and their families are being pushed forward, it is clear that we need many more people to take an interest in mental health.

One must also emphasize the need for much more research into mental disease, its causes and its treatment. Britain gets praise in other countries for its free and continuing service and its interlocked system of doctors and psychiatric social workers, but also because it employs in the NHS a great variety of techniques and allows its specialists to cover quite a wide range of theories as to cause and treatment. There is a considerable conflict between those who advocate and use physical means, for example, convulsive therapy and, increasingly, drugs affecting the whole nervous and mental systems; and those who use only psychological techniques, which are often time-consuming and apply in some cases to the individual, in others to a group. Much more has to be done in studying the epidemiology of mental disease, and in emphasizing the community angle of this problem; the whole health team must be involved in the study of one of man's most pressing problems.

There is, of course, a National Association for Mental Health, which watches what is happening to patients in British mental hospitals and has influenced much of the change in attitudes of the public and of hospital staff. One of the Association's most active propagandists, Christopher Mayhew, MP, has said, on this question of studying the epidemiology of mental illness, that 'if only schizophrenia had been infective like polio we would have seen a drive to get on top of the problem'. Mr Mayhew and some of his colleagues have spent nights in mental hospital wards in order to see exactly what went on. They were not so horrified as might have been expected, but hope that the kind of knowledge they gained will rouse public feeling on the subject.

One part of that arousal is persuading people that they can help the mentally sick by keeping them at home and using the hospital facilities for daytime care, or by taking lonely people with minor mental illness into their homes as lodgers but treating them as members of the family. A group of doctors working in Melrose, Scotland, have described in *The Lancet* (8 January 1972) how they aim not to treat mental disease as if it was like other illnesses that can be 'cured' by drugs. They believe that 'except for periods of the most acute stress or psychosis, admission to hospital may be unnecessary and even therapeutically undesirable'. They would like to see the money being made available used to provide much more accommodation of the hostel type, with a really 'radical revision of modern psychiatric planning'. With so many views of mental health being put forward, with so much needing to be spent in any case in improved accommodation, such replanning would seem to match most of the thinking on the development of the NHS in the next two decades.

Chapter 15

Occupational Health

Modern industry is full of inherent health problems but it continually develops new ones within its various organizations, and inflicts hazards upon the population outside. The health history of industry in all modern societies is one of very bad beginnings and a long struggle to remove the worst abuses—child labour, long hours, dangerous procedures. The study of occupational disease began in 1700 with the publication in Italy of the works of Ramazzini who had studied the health of a great number of workers in different trades and found few who were not adversely affected. He wanted to create interest among other physicians who would also study the subject and assist in obtaining 'a really complete and thorough treatise worthy of a place in the department of medicine. At any rate we owe this to the wretched condition of the workers from whose manual toil, so necessary though sometimes very mean and sordid, so many benefits accrue to the commonwealth of mankind.' Much of industry, in spite of his exposures, was to remain mean and sordid for another 200 years, and even today there are industrial processes in modern societies which are still hazardous; and in developing countries the first stages of industrial growth are still accompanied by dangers and disease. They are complicated also by the same nutritional deficiencies and infections of various kinds that made the industries of the nineteenth century in European countries so destructive of life. At that time there was no scientific knowledge of infections or of the effects of dietary deficiencies, but reformers did realize that dirt, filth and poverty were all parts of the problem and sought to get rid of these. The work of the early social reformers was beginning to improve conditions when the discovery of bacteria and, later, the recognition of definite deficiencies in certain elements of diet, confirmed the validity of much that had been written about the health of the workers. Today, René Dubos says, 'one has only to contrast the sickly proletariat described by Engels and the tall husky men now typical of the working classes in prosperous Western countries to appreciate what miracles can be wrought in a short time'. True: but it must not make us disregard the dangers inside industry and created by it.

Nor must we conclude that the overall effect of poverty on health has disappeared from our industrial workers and their families. In April 1970 the Secretary of State estimated there were 110,000 families of men in full-time work who were below what he considered the poverty line, and others estimate that the figure was and remains much higher. The National Food Surveys have shown in the past ten years that low income groups with both parents and three or four children fall well below the levels recommended by the BMA for the intake of protein and calcium. We no longer have the tragic amount of rickets among children that was a feature of industrial areas, but whenever poverty, and especially the poverty of the unemployed, prevents the adequate consumption of foodstuffs containing vitamin D, the medical profession has to be on the alert against the return of this now unfamiliar disease. The NHS has made possible the diagnosis and treatment of disease; but unless industry ensures wages high enough to ensure adequate nutrition, preventable ill health will still occur. It may be minor in nature but that is something industry should be anxious to avoid, for no worker can give of his best if his health is below normal.

Britain is now so industrialized that the total environment can be adversely affected by industrial processes. There is the whole question of pollution—of the air by fumes, of the rivers and sea by industrial effluents and by the necessity to get rid of waste material, which has led to the scandal and danger of dumping of industrial poisons. Cyanide, as the public now knows, is used in various industrial processes and although known to be a deadly poison has been dumped in large quantities in a very dangerous fashion. The efforts now being made to give us clean air are having effects all can see; and if industry can be compelled not to put poisons into our rivers we will have greatly improved water supplies and possibilities of fishing. When we speak of doctors needing to have a sense of social responsibility even more than any other group of citizens we include among the problems on which they have to express themselves as experts in health this whole field of industrial damage to the environment.

Within industry there are two main health questions still to be tackled. The first has long had official recognition: the question of safety within industry. There has been a gradual realization of the danger of accidents when men are handling powerful tools, tools for cutting, for crushing, for rapid processing of metal, and so on; and the need for studying every process and providing safeguards is accepted by all. But manufacturers have often been reluctant to carry out the necessary modifications to machines and processes because they slow up production; and workmen do not always carry out their part of the safety code if it makes production more difficult or slower. There have been many Acts of Parliament to improve safeguards and the Chief Factory Inspector in his annual reports continually stresses that in spite of all efforts accidents go on increasing.

The total number of casualties and their effect on industry are seldom appreciated. John Taylor, writing for World Health Day in April 1969 drew attention to the estimates of the International Labour Office that in World War II 'British forces suffered casualties, including dead, at the rate of nearly 11,000 a month. In factories in Britain, casualties were at the same time running at over 22,000 a month'. War, of course, made the risk of casualties in factories working at high speed abnormally high but in 1970 factory accidents topped 300,000. Experience in the USA was the same—casualties in the armed forces about 25,000 a month, in American factories over 160,000 a month'. But illness is just as serious or even more so for in the UK 'the illness rate per week is, according to the industry, nine to fourteen times higher than the accident rate'. In Britain in recent years 'for every minute lost through labour disputes, nine minutes were lost through industrial injuries and over two hours through sickness. One German worker in ten has an accident each year. In the US over 500 million working days are lost annually because of illness.'

Table 15.1 gives the figures of recorded accidents since the NHS

Table 15.1. Casualties in Industry

Year	*Fatal*	*Non-fatal*	*Total*
1948	552	182,286	182,838
1952	471	154,995	155,466
1963	610	203,659	204,269
1966	701	295,909	296,610
1969	668	321,622	322,390

came into being but does not indicate how severe the accidents have been or how much of a burden their treatment has put on the hospital service. Nor does this table indicate the long-term result of many accidents. Under the Industrial Injuries Act very large numbers of injured are paid short-term benefits but in 1966 there were 120,000 people receiving life disablement benefits. Other figures hint at how much incapacity results from injuries which are called accidents but could almost all be prevented if proper action were taken.

The story is the same in other countries. All industrial countries now have rules, regulations and laws about factory safety, and some have quite advanced services for those injured at work. There are few statistics as to the degree of risk in different factories but one interesting study in Chicago has shown that the risk can be very high. In 1968 the survey showed that only in 20 per cent of the plants examined was there no evident occupational health hazard, while 73 per cent 'had at least one employee at risk to toxic materials'. The survey writers considered that in 72 per cent of the plants there were adequate safeguards for only half the workers and there appeared to be at least 100 different physical, chemical or other hazardous agents. The survey also noted that apart from actual hazards, more than half the plants, employing 43 per cent of the in-plant workers, had unacceptably bad sanitary conditions, what may be described as bad housekeeping, and were dangerous to health. Poor lighting and ventilation are very common, and noise is a hazard in many industries.

One country which claims to be tackling all these problems is the Soviet Union, which has a very large amount of legislation dealing with the protection of the worker. It is claimed that the design of both machinery and factories is looked at from the health angle at every stage so that safeguards can be built into the system. To a considerable extent automated processes are used in which the machines are under control from a distance, and this is seen as one way to cut down accidents. But there are also in every factory experts in safety and in improving conditions of work, who co-operate with committees of workers to ensure that rules are obeyed. There is in every factory in the USSR an annual negotiated agreement, made between management and trade unions, and such agreements usually contain clauses setting out the health problems that have to be tackled and allocating funds for all that can be considered as conducive to health, better sanitation, ventilation and lighting, and for education on the whole subject of avoidable industrial risks.

The second main health question in industry includes but also goes far beyond the avoidance of hazards and the treatment of accidents when they occur: the provision of a comprehensive Occupational Health Service (OHS). All who suffer from industrial injury, poisoning at work and so on receive care from the various units of the NHS. But this is not enough. The complexities covered by 'health service at work' require something else, not a separate service but a fully developed service integrated with the new NHS. It has of course to go on treating the things that do happen to workers;

but it has to move into new fields. First the job of preventing hazards must be prosecuted with the utmost vigour. With our present technological abilities it should be a criminal offence for any factory or undertaking to continue with processes or use machinery which has inherent dangers. But since education, prevention and rehabilitation are all involved, the workers individually and collectively must be brought into the control of the service. On the accident prevention side safety committees must be compulsory and must allow for adequate worker participation. The medical and safety officers serving such a committee must be able to act, and must be seen to act, quite independently of management. Of course in an integrated health service the doctors would be full-time employees of the NHS and so could act quite independently in all health matters. It must not be thought, however, that such a committee or such a service would be inimical to the employers. The forerunner of the Confederation of British Industry once said that an occupational health service provided by employers themselves but using the facilities of the NHS would, among other things, 'provide immediate treatment for medical and surgical emergencies and minor illnesses at work; provide "follow up" treatment at work (and so save production time); collaborate with the worker's GP; help persons returning after a period of illness to settle back into the working routine; examine applicants for jobs as to their health and help management to avoid hazards to health and to maintain healthy working conditions.' All this, it was seen, would save production time and help everyone towards a healthier life.

For the Trades Union Congress this declaration did not go far enough and it certainly does not approach the need for a comprehensive service; one that to begin with, at least, would establish priorities so that services were first started where they were most needed and irrespective of whether the industries with the greatest need were the ones that would make the biggest contribution to the OHS funds. (It was then and still is thought that to finance the OHS within the NHS would require additional contributions from employers.) But the TUC wanted to go much further. The service they wanted must not be mainly curative, it must protect workers against all hazards, and this would mean 'making a close study of the risks to health that arise from conditions of work as well as the condition of the worker'. This is a very important point, one constantly reiterated in the literature of the Soviet Union and acted on in its factories: dangers to health must be eliminated but 'physical fitness must be ensured'. The point the TUC wants to emphasize is that it is one thing to establish a good industrial environment; it is also necessary to find the right and fit worker for every job. It follows that 'to improve industrial efficiency and safeguard health . . . an occupational health service must make use of specialised techniques in ergonomics and medicine far beyond the scope of a medical officer appointed to deal with minor injuries and illnesses'.

The problem now to be faced is how to link with the NHS and above all with the family doctor, who certifies sickness for benefit purposes, a group of doctors and nurses trained in industrial health, and to give them security of position so that they can feel independent and so that they can co-operate with the workers, who must be actively involved in all these questions. The latest Act of Parliament makes the setting up of safety committees in places employing more than 100 people compulsory, 'to promote co-operation between management and workers for achieving and maintaining safe and healthy working conditions'. Safety is less a medical problem than one for management and the designers and makers of machinery; but every machine and every process needs medical study. Industry has done some work in this field, but so little has been properly applied that the Trades Union Congress has had to step into this field and in conjunction with the London School of Hygiene has established an advisory service and laboratories where certain research is being carried out. The TUC has long had its own medical adviser but has never had to seek medical service for trade unionists, as has been the case in the USA. The TUC, however, is in agreement with the Labour Party, to which nearly all the trade unions are also affiliated, that an occupational health service must be the next big development in health care in Britain.

One factor must influence thinking on this subject, the number of small factories in the country. Even if all factories were big enough to have a staffed medical centre within their gates a close link between the doctors of the factory environment and the doctors of the community would be essential. In Britain, with a quarter of a million work-places far too small to have medical or nursing staff always on the premises, a practical working collaboration, and indeed overlap of personnel and services, is essential. Among other things that must not be overlooked is the fact that 'it is work which gives a man his status and place in the community and is thus a major factor in his state of health'. The writers quoted, Dr Frank Tyrer of Rochdale Industrial Health Service and Dr Robert Murray, TUC Medical Adviser, went on (*The Lancet*, 24 August 1968): 'In this field the distinction between the effects of work on health and of health on work becomes blurred—they mesh like the teeth of two great wheels revolving in a vicious circle.' Such a concept clearly ties together the community health team and the OHS doctors, but must also involve the active involvement of the citizens as patients and workers. Tyrer and Murray continue: 'Here lies the area for the next great advances in occupational medicine, which will be more hardly won than the triumphs over the physical environment—but they cannot be made by doctors alone.'

In the next stage of development of health care, therefore, all aspects of occupational health must be included and integrated with the other existing services. In few places will it be necessary or even advisable for Britain to build new hospitals to deal with accidents of industry, although in many places bigger and better emergency departments will be needed. Once the clear responsibility of a district hospital to deal with industrial accidents is established the staffing will have to be reconsidered with this in mind. Anyone who has seen the kind of special institutes for dealing with accidental trauma in countries like Italy and the USSR will realize that good as some of our units are, all hospitals near heavy industry will have to be better equipped than they are today. In the smaller factories, and apart from accidents, the doctors will need to have a place of work, and one which brings them into close contact with the family doctors; in other words, occupational health must be one of the functions of the health centres. This is no new idea. Writing in *Medicine Today and Tomorrow* (May 1952), Dr Frank Tyrer, from his own experience as an industrial medical officer, said: 'Workers are tending more and more to consult their works doctors and nurses about all kinds of personal and even family problems which in theory are the province of the NHS.' He thought that a few of the better services already provided by employers in some industries had created the idea of a fusion of preventive and curative medical services of which the 'culmination must be the nation-wide provision of health centres on which the factory medical services covering groups of small works, as well as the general practitioner services, shall be based'. Today more than ever the time has come for a great acceleration of the building of health centres which will enable such a service to begin.

Health centres as presently envisaged may not be able to tackle an aspect of occupational health which is one of our greater lacks at present: full rehabilitation and retraining services. These are not the same thing. Rehabilitation is needed for all whose muscles have been weakened by illness or injury. We have not taken the subject sufficiently seriously in this country. We certainly do not give convalescence therapy anything like the place it is given in the Soviet Union. There full use is made of their spas and watering-places by a system integral with health care but administered by the trade unions. Retraining should mean the training for new kinds of work of men and women who, because of injury or disease, ought not to return to the same factory and the same job in case they should meet the same hazard again. This is a field in which the doctors of the OHS and the family doctors must co-operate to assess both the man and the job; and if they no longer fit (or perhaps never fitted), to see that the man is trained in some suitable work. One of the things that must be stressed is that ability to do a worthwhile job is man's chief sign to himself and others that he is healthy and well.

It will be argued that we have not enough doctors with the necessary skills, and it may be that in some health centres and in some places some of the GPs will need to do, as many have done in the past, some work within industry. But they will need training and above all will have to learn the new work that has to be done in industry. As Tyrer and Murray put it: 'If the notion that work is a healthful activity, with a therapeutic value at the right stage of convalescence, is correct, every effort must be made, in conjunction with rather than opposition to the family doctor, to prevent the unnecessary prolongation of absence under cover of a medical certificate.' For half a century Britain's GPs have been undertaking the task of certifying fitness and non-fitness for work. In conjunction with the industrial doctors, working in the same health centres, this task would be better done with the onus shared by someone who really understood the job the man or woman did.

We must not, however, talk of factories as though they were the only places in which people work. Offices, schools, shops and all kinds of institutions must be covered, since in all these there are health hazards and problems. Agriculture is an industry which needs more and more medical attention, for it is now both a mechanical and a chemical industry that has, by its rural nature, not always had the medical care it needs. There are, too, the great problems of providing healthy food, the obverse of the story of pollution, and the more doctors we have connected with agriculture and linked with veterinary scientists, the better chance we should have of ensuring food for the people. Nor must we overlook the industry which employs more women than all the others together: looking after the home. As places of work tens of thousands of houses are as badly equipped and planned as the worst factory; and injury and even death are all too common. Our arrangements to deal with emergencies in the industry of housekeeping are as poor as in many small factories. The health centres as they come along must be staffed with this also in mind. Just as injured men and women need a great deal of help to get back to work, so the woman in the home must have the same attention. Every doctor, and every citizen, must also be aware that houses can be designed for the crippled, the disabled and the elderly. None of these should live in a house they cannot enter without going up steps; and doors should be wide enough for the wheelchairs now needed, and used, by thousands of people.

Finally we must not overlook that the health industry has its hazards and dangers, and doctors and nurses are not the best people at looking after themselves. They begin their careers as students and the whole educational and medical industries between them merit and need an occupationally orientated health care system. The education of the doctor in all these aspects of prevention could very well start with young people in training.

Chapter 16

Aid between Countries

Health care and a general interest in health itself should be a unifying force not only within a single country, as we have suggested earlier, but between nations. Indeed, those organs of the United Nations which are most concerned with health or with its procurement, with agricultural organization, with the care of children, have been most successful in getting international co-operation. The International Labour Office, which concerns itself to a large extent with the health of the workers, has also achieved remarkable co-operation among nations; and the World Health Organization is probably the most completely co-operative and internationally accepted of organizations. That co-operation does not always produce as much money for international schemes as its officers and advocates think it should have; but its work is appreciated in most countries of the world. Health is even included in treaties between nations, for both the Treaty of Rome, establishing the European Common Market, and the North Atlantic Treaty Organization (NATO), include arrangements for the future development of common health services. They recognize, in an imperfect way, that rapid and easy movement of people must mean co-operation to preserve the world's health, but also that individuals need health protection wherever they go. Health protection includes requirements by most countries that visitors must have been immunized against certain diseases; it further implies that countries having large numbers of overseas visitors must also watch out against the importation of infectious disease; and this may include animals as well as humans. So there has to be a great deal of co-operation between countries, most of it organized through WHO. One very large part of that co-operation concerns the collection of health statistics and it is on WHO reports that most people comparing the health records of different nations depend.

There is in fact no aspect of health which is not of international importance. It is one thing to try to prevent the spread of infectious diseases by immunizing and checking upon travellers. It is clearly even more important to get at places where infectious diseases are usually endemic and by assisting the local people try to rid the world of a dangerous disease. The World Health Organization has launched and managed big campaigns to rid countries, and ultimately the world, of malaria, smallpox and so on, and with considerable success. At the same time experts and expertise are offered to underdeveloped countries in their struggle to upgrade their health care, and WHO has urged the richer nations to give money as well as other forms of aid. Such aid is now a very important part of international agreements and goes far beyond medical aid, but in the health field there have been many successes. In the educational field also there has been aid and some success, and educational aid has included help in medical education. We have seen how affluent countries have been considering or are actually engaged in training special medical aids as one way of overcoming the shortage of doctors, which is universal, and this has been a special interest of WHO. That organization has held many conferences on the need for the poorer countries to develop a basic health unit which, under medical supervision, could give rudimentary but scientific help to rural populations. What it proposed was that countries should be advised on what could be accepted as a minimum standard of adequate service, a network of linked peripheral and central units, 'staffed by competent professional and auxiliary personnel and capable of performing effectively a selected group of functions essential to the health of the people living in an area'. It should be noted that they hoped for a selected group of functions, not patients. Some years later a WHO Technical Report (No. 472, 1971) declared: 'It seems clear that health services will be organized to meet the needs of entire populations and not merely of selected groups. The entire population, both the sick and the healthy, will need to be able to call on services for the protection and maintenance of health as well as a full range of preventive curative and rehabilitative services'.

The problem of doing so is both financial and technical, and a full study of its difficulties will be found in *Health and the Developing World* (1969), a Rockefeller Foundation report by Dr John Bryant. In his preface to the book he says: 'Large numbers of the world's people, perhaps more than half, have no access to health care at all and for many of the rest the care they receive does not answer the problems they have'. The application of medical science is a universal problem, for the task of providing care 'is difficult in Malawi, one of the world's poorest countries, and so is it difficult in the United States, one of the world's richest'. In a very telling table, partly quoted in Table 16.1 he indicates the range between the

Table 16.1 Indicators of National Development and Health[1]

Country	*Population mid-1965 (millions)*	*GNP per capita (US$)*	*Annual g'ment expenditure on health (per capita, US$)*	*Population per doctor*	*Population per hospital bed*
Malawi	3.9	40	0.64	145,000	940
Sudan	13.5	95	1.02	29,000	990
Thailand	30.59	120	1.77	2,800	520
Colombia	18.07	260	3.50	2,000	320
Sweden	7.73	2,130	88.00	960	70

1 Adapted from Table 17, *Health and the Developing World* (1969), John Bryant.

really poor and the affluent. These figures are comparable, and the comparison stands, but they are for 1965 or nearest year. In a paper in *WHO Chronicle* (December 1971), Benjamin gives some later figures contrasting Ethiopia, with 65,000 people per doctor and a per capita income of $55; India, with 4,800 and $90; Chile, with 2,320 and $480; the USSR, with 450 and $1,000; and the US itself with 1,080 and $3,240.

When Bryant discusses further the educational problems involved in trying to provide the whole health team out of societies still largely illiterate, he reaches a conclusion the rest of the world must heed. 'The great unmet health need, the serious deficiencies in systems for health care and the most telling educational inadequacies —these cluster around the single but painfully complex question of how to provide care for large numbers of people on limited resources'. Since all the nations which are members of WHO are committed to the search for a healthy world, these limited resources will need a great deal of support and even then it is doubtful whether the impoverished parts of the world will come anywhere near the standards of the developed countries this century.

If we were to turn to another aspect of health, nutrition, we would find exactly the same large question looming not only over those countries which are poor at present, but over the whole world: can the expected population of AD 2,000 be fed even if all the proposals for increasing the food supply of the earth are carried out? The pessimists who think we will not curb the population increase rapidly enough to ensure a sufficient food supply certainly appear to have the better of statistical arguments. So far as vast populations – the whole of India, much of Africa and of South-East Asia – are concerned, malnutrition is already the rule and the ill health that goes with malnutrition afflicts millions of people. This intensifies everything one has to say about the need for perfecting ways of delivering health care, for the complete removal of financial barriers to health care throughout the world, and for the setting up of an international agreement on how health care is to be given to all the world's citizens.

The basis must be that all scientific medical knowledge that any country has must be available to all. Nutrition we know about. We know fairly well what people require for health; we can calculate the world needs of the basic foodstuffs, essential elements such as vitamins; and we can educate people in the better use of what food there is or will be. Population increase we also know about. We can calculate how many people will inhabit the earth in the immediate future: and we know it is essential that man reduces his birth rate if population is to decrease and the human race survive. We know also that high birth rates accompany poverty and illiteracy, often backed by religious beliefs which over the centuries have done little to attack these great flaws in man's development. The whole world needs more and better information on family planning; and the medical men and women of all countries will be lacking in social responsibility if they do not join in the continuous education of their patients on the subject. It must be made clear to the impoverished that not only do too many children increase poverty, but the great improvements in child care mean that the survival of children is now so much better that no one needs, as they once did, to have a lot of children so that one may survive.

Beyond these simpler aspects of human health there are many questions to be faced as to what man can do or will do about his own evolution. The forces that moulded man operated over millions of years and evolution was a very long process. Does the modern urban way of life inhibit further evolution, and if so has man the scientific knowledge to modify his own genetic structure so as to manipulate man's further evolution along lines worked out by man himself? It is still doubtful to what extent man can change his own genetics, but if he has this potential then scientists and doctors who embark on it must have very full understanding of what is involved and must not claim independence from the control of ordinary people just because the latter do not have the technical knowledge.

Meantime man must press on with the other principle which flows from the acceptance of health as a human right, the provision of health care on an international basis. If medicine is to be taken out of the market-place then no qualified medical man should ever use the plight of a foreign visitor to his own country as an excuse for making large, and even extortionate sums of money out of the sick of other lands—and for many reasons. First there is the general ethical reason that one does not make a profit from the misfortune of others even if one has a skill they urgently need. Secondly, the highest medical ethic that can be attained is to give a gift to a stranger, and especially the gift of health or life itself. Thirdly, when one provides wealthy foreigners with a service they could not get in their own country, and have made no political effort to provide there, privilege is being emphasised and the desire for privilege used as a means of making a profit. Why should the poor of an underdeveloped country have not even basic care while their rulers or aristocracy can come to Britain for forms of health care provided by the taxpayer and public resources?

It might have been argued in the past that there was something fine, even to be praised, in a British surgeon helping a visitor who needed surgery even if he was asked for a lot of money. But the exploitation of Britain's reformed abortion laws has shown just what can happen. Thousands of abortions, probably one-third of the total, have been done for foreign women outside the NHS hospitals by practitioners who have apparently made very large amounts of money in this way. Because this item of medical care was and is a profitable one in the market-place the desired aim of making necessary abortions possible has been brought into some disrepute. The Birmingham Pregnancy Advisory Service has said, as reported in *The Times* (8 March 1972, that 'the abortion market stood out from other private health field activities. It provided exceptional opportunities for quick money-making, springing from the patient's urgent need, helplessness and ignorance. This attracted not only some doctors and providers of nursing homes, but an unusual number of intermediaries and touts, rarely found in other branches of medicine.' The voluntary Birmingham advisory body thought that this is a field in which public intervention to control the service is essential. It is not this form of international traffic that one is recommending in speaking of international health care for the individual. As Professor Maurice King, writing from Zambia, has put it (*The Lancet*, 25 March 1972), the motto of doctors everywhere should be: 'It is our business to see that no man shall want for what medicine might readily do'.

The British NHS has been of great service to many hundreds of foreign visitors who have become sick or had an accident while in the British Isles. Those who come here to work have the right to choose a doctor just like any other worker and of course they pay their taxes and so make a contribution to the national budget which pays for the NHS. The people who have had the greatest benefit are the tourists who have suddenly found themselves in a British hospital and, especially Americans, begin to wonder what they will have to pay only to find there is no charge. Anyone visiting the USA from Britain will be told story after story about how wonderful British medical care is and how remarkable it is that no money is asked for by anyone. It is in fact one of the greatest recommendations the NHS gets. It was a deliberate decision that 'health for all' means what it says, and that Britain's gift to any sick person is the care he needs. Naturally some people have protested against this use of taxpayers' money, but no one has seriously suggested altering it. In twenty years many Chancellors have looked at the question, found that the grand total involved was not very much in relation to a national service, and that it would cost more to set up a machine for collecting the money – and chasing after bad debts – than would ever be collected. It is now established and recognized all over the world as a step towards a system of international health care.

Britain is, however, not unique. The USSR provides visitors with medical care exactly as Britain does and although up to the present there are not so many tourists in the Soviet Union as in some other countries the number is growing, and many people have had the service of Russian doctors and hospitals. Britain and the USSR have not exchanged any agreement on this subject for both do the same for their visitors. But the UK has tried to enlarge on its own arrangements by making reciprocal agreements with other countries.

Reciprocity is, of course, difficult since so few countries have a service and must depend on sick funds to finance at least primary care and in some cases, hospital care and doctors' fees. It follows that all a country with which Britain makes an agreement can do is to guarantee to a British subject who needs care that he or she will get no less than the citizens of the country concerned. Reciprocity can apply to more than health care. As we have seen, in most countries health care is part of an overall social security system. There has been in recent years a considerable advance in making social security benefits portable so that 'persons who move from one country to another either keep the social security rights acquired in the first country or have them replaced by corresponding rights in the other country'. Because of the variations, however, it is not possible to make the same reciprocal arrangements with all the countries which are prepared to reach agreement. Britain has agreements with twenty-six countries covering as few as two benefits and as many as eleven.

In health, comprehensive reciprocal plans have been made with only six countries, Bulgaria, Denmark, New Zealand, Norway, Sweden and Yugoslavia. With another seven countries the arrangements are restricted and apply only to people 'resident' in the country concerned and vice versa. With all the rest only money arrangements are possible but at least the principle of making such reciprocal arrangements as are possible has been established. As countries develop more complete services, more such agreements can be reached.

The position is even more interesting among the European countries, for under the Treaty of Rome members of the European Economic Community should have already reached agreement on some kind of common health service and should have complete interchange of social service schemes. The motivating point for this is that the EEC postulates free movement of workers among the present six member countries. If Britain and others go in such reciprocity will have to be extended. Britain already has agreement on exchange of social service benefits with all the six but no agreement on health care. Denmark and Norway apart from the EEC already have agreements on health with each other and Britain, but also with Sweden, Finland and Iceland. There will clearly be many things to negotiate within an extended Common Market and the UK will have to be very firm that it will make reciprocal agreements but will not go back to an insurance system, however complete.

The concept has, moreover, to be extended still further, for under the NATO agreement at some point in time there should be a common health scheme for citizens of all the NATO countries. These include Canada and the US, the former with its new national health system, the latter still seeking one; and also Portugal, Turkey and Greece, which could not offer a service comparable to that available in other NATO countries except by giving the visitors from these countries special attention. In all three countries hospital care is largely government financed and good services could be made available at the largest hospitals. Switzerland, which receives so many tourists, has its own form of health insurance, which does not very closely resemble any of the others, but on social services has very comprehensive agreements with Britain. It is possible that to meet all the present variations it would be best if each country made health care a portable right, as Canada has done, so that in those countries which had no international understandings the citizen requiring attention could send the bill to his own government.

There are two further aspects of the problem that overlap between developed and not yet modernized states, the position of the Church and the position of research. It will be recalled that the Church, of all denominations of the Christian faith but also of many other religions, has had a part to play in the provision of health care. In the European countries, and in territories which they controlled overseas, the Church from earliest times has provided some services that were partly social and partly medical in their functions. Today in most Western societies the Churches still own medical institutions and as we have seen in Belgium, Portugal and Spain a high proportion of hospital beds are controlled by religious bodies. In Britain, when the old poor-law and the voluntary hospitals were united a decision was made that religious institutions should remain outside the NHS. Today they are nearly all outside but make contractual arrangements to sell beds to the national service. On the Continent that decision has not been necessary although as the State or sick funds pay most of the costs even the most religious institution has to fit into the national plan.

In underdeveloped countries as many as 40 per cent of hospital beds are provided by religious bodies, a high proportion being missionary organizations. Bryant (in *Health and the Developing World*) estimates there are 3,000 such bodies with an operating budget of over $300 million annually. In India one finds excellent hospitals – Anglican, Presbyterian, Roman Catholic and Hundi – all providing a high quality of care but almost entirely within the hospital field and largely specialist in nature. The contribution is, therefore, considerable, but there is a change in many countries for the question has been raised as to whether, faced with greatly increased costs and with their own inability to do more than tackle a small part of ascertained ill health, this is still a job for religious people. They see that what is needed is a comprehensive service and this they can never supply; while many doubt the relevance of supplying pockets of hospital care through trained (and not necessarily religious) staffs.

Research is vital to any health service not only because new discoveries are important, but because it requires and attracts men and women of active minds who make their special contribution to any medical institution in which they work. Research may be done in special laboratories, divorced from ordinary routine work, but in all countries a great deal of basic research is done in hospital laboratories, and all clinical research must by its nature be done in clinical institutions. In the underdeveloped countries the cost of modern research makes the building up of research staffs a matter of great difficulty, and yet agencies which give aid to such countries have to beware of giving equipment which cannot be serviced or maintained, or may even not be economically used because there is no one available with the skill that is needed.

In Western countries quite an amount of money is spent on research in highly developed laboratories in medical schools, universities and large hospitals, and a considerable amount is spent by chemical and drug firms. In his *International Study of Health Expenditures* (1967), B. Abel-Smith gives figures for many countries but does not separate teaching and research, which are in fact often closely linked. Australia, Canada, Ceylon, Finland, Yugoslavia and the United Kingdom all show figures of between 2.5 and 3.0 per cent of the total indirect expenditure on health services, the high spenders being Poland (5.2 per cent,) the Netherlands (8.2 per cent) and the USA (8.8 per cent). The latter country has gone on spending very large amounts on medical research. Rice and Cooper (*Bulletin of Social Security Administration*, January 1972) give the figure for the fiscal year 1970–1 as $2,019 million, but that does not include the amount spent by drug houses. In Britain it is estimated that over £100 million is spent on research and development, of which between £25 million and £30 million is laid out by the pharmaceutical industry. A similar amount is spent in universities and that is mainly on basic scientific research. Many voluntary organisations, and hospitals from their own funds, spend money on clinical research, but the bulk of the money directly applied to medical research comes from the £20 million funds of the Medical Research Council. It has its own laboratories and other institutions, but also distributes funds, for specified research projects, to many NHS laboratories and hospitals. There is a moderate amount of money donated by grateful patients and relatives directly to laboratories they want to help, but this is not a large proportion of the money available within the health service. There is a scheme for the encouragement of research which is initiated locally and to this allocations amounting to approximately £750,000 are made. Regional hospital boards control these allocations and add their own from their own endowment funds. Of all the spendings within the NHS that on research is probably the one on which reaching an agreement as to what is a fair amount would be most difficult. What is essential is not so much that large sums are offered for research on specified subjects, like the American spending on cancer and cardio-vascular disease, but that money should be readily available when a promising line of research opens up. When money is not freely available then research tends to fall behind those sections of the health care system which have a more immediate clinical application. The public in Britain can always be stimulated to give money when someone appears to be being treated unfairly. That spirit needs to be translated into a readiness to see more public money made available in every one of the new health districts that are proposed, so that the whole service feels the impact of research and is ready to develop and apply new ideas.

There is one further aspect of co-operation in international health, that of standardization of materials used in medicine and of units of measurement used in examinations of the body, its tissues and fluids. Various bodies are interested in this, the Council of Europe, for example, as well as WHO and ad hoc organizations. The International Committee for Standardization in Haematology, for example, is putting forward a whole list of new units based on the metric system, because 'it is essential for haematological practice to conform to the practices of related specialities and for any change which is contemplated to be agreed upon nationally and internationally in order to avoid confusion and unfamiliarity which could lead to lethal misunderstanding'. There are many other fields in which international units will be necessary, and all of this is part of the build-up of that common volume of medical knowledge which may ultimately lead, as some believe, to a World Health Service. The concept has been well expressed by Dr G. E. W. Wolstenholme in *Health of Mankind* (Ciba Foundation, 1967), where he speaks of a 'healthy fraternity of nations'. Once the idea of the WHS was established, 'the recruitment of all members of the WHS would be expected to establish standards for the world as a whole. To be selected would be an affair of pride, and to have served in the WHS a recommendation for one's future career'. No one who has considered the work of WHO, and who has studied the principles we have discussed here as to how medicine can really satisfy the right to health, can doubt that 'the forces of sickness, injury and infirmity face us with a worthy and a shaming challenge . It is a challenge the health workers of the world will certainly have to meet.

Chapter 17

Education

If research epitomizes the spirit of a modern health care system, education in all its aspects is the basis on which both the quantity and the quality of the medical attention to be given to the people depend. When we write of 'all its aspects' we refer to more than the straightforward education of the medical student. His education is changing rapidly, and to the end of this century must be a very flexible affair. But we have to go on to discuss his continuing education, for there is universal agreement that all doctors must be given fresh information on new techniques and methods so long as they deal with patients. But the wider aspects may be even more important, the parallel education and re-education of all health workers. Whether they are in close contact with the physician or work in an independent capacity it is essential that their knowledge should also cover all new discoveries and new ideas.

Two other elements of education are also important, that of the non-professional workers in the health service and that of the general public. The former should know the general strategy for health, what it means in training, what kind of clinical considerations must influence administration and planning. As for the general public, their education must also be continuous and must not only cover individual health, and that at different ages, but must include some general education in hygiene and in health measures that affect the population as a whole. How much of this education should be part of school teaching and how much of it should come later it is probably not necessary to discuss, for both must go on. But adults must be taught to relate health to the community in which they live.

Popular education in health in most countries has been made more difficult than it need be by two factors: doctors are trained and paid to look after the sick, and they have no duty to teach their own or any other patients. In a country like the UK where 'advertising' is prohibited and even talking to a public audience, or writing a popular book, may be considered to be advertising, doctors are actively prevented from attempting public education. It is true that Britain has an official Health Education Council and public health doctors, and the Department of Health give public instruction in many ways. But what is needed is involvement of the people and the doctors in a joint effort to establish good health and to prevent disease. What is done in Britain is not nearly vigorous enough or continuous enough, and the advertising and sale of 'patent medicines' not only works against the creation of health, for it postulates ill health, but uses the advertising media in a way that illustrates what could be done if we really wanted to educate the people.

One probably sees the greatest contrast in this field in the USSR where there is a separate Ministry for Health Education, and much money is spent on health propaganda. The system has its weaknesses, for while there is no advertising of cigarettes there is little propaganda against smoking. But health education begins at birth. The child is immediately attached to a children's polyclinic, where he will be both looked after and exhorted to follow a healthy way of life. *The System of Public Health Services in the USSR* (1967) says: 'The successful solution of many of the problems connected with the protection and improvement of the people's health is possible only if the entire population and various public organizations are drawn into public health work'. Every doctor in the USSR is expected to carry out regular health education in the community in which he works, and every health establishment has a Council of Voluntary Public Service which enrols people from the community to assist actively in sanitary and hygienic campaigns. There is a 'Health Day' annually during which the work of the health services is thrown open to public discussion and display. But health is also carried into the factories where 'exercise periods', during which the workers do special exercises to keep them fit, are very popular. It is claimed they improve production as well as health. The whole of the spa form of convalescence includes physical exercise and instruction on keeping fit.

There is no advertising of medicines in the USSR, although home remedies can be purchased at pharmacies. There is indeed quite an amount of self-treatment, as there is in all countries, but it is not subject to the spurious or vociferous public claims such as most other countries experience. Self-medication has of course existed down the ages, and at one time used herbs and other substances man had found to have beneficial effects. Unfortunately, as C. D. Leake said in *Home Medication and the Public Welfare* (New York Academy of Sciences, 1965), 'with the rise of modern technology and particularly with the development of current advertising methods, people have been persuaded to purchase useless or, unfortunately, sometimes dangerous drugs or drug combinations for their own use'. The selling of drugs direct to people must be one of the factors which has led to the growing abuse of addictive drugs. The amount of some medicaments now being sold is measured in tons and in millions of tablets. H. George Mandel, in the book on home medication already quoted, gives some fascinating figures for the United States. The most startling concern aspirin: in 1963 there were more than 1,000 brands of aspirin preparations being sold, 28 million pounds' weight in all.

The whole subject of proprietary remedies sold to the public is vast. The point to be made here is that the inculcation of the habit of self-medication which in itself and with simple remedies – there are few 'safe' remedies if we look at the list of accidental poisonings – is harmless, even useful, leads to many false ideas on both health and disease. The new medium, television, does incalculable harm to all ideas of creating a healthy public through an understanding of basic health principles. Even if the Department of Health took up as much time as is spent on advertising drugs, cigarettes and alcohol on television screens, and as much space in newspapers and magazines, it would be a difficult task to counter all the false claims and suggestive points relating these three potentially addictive substances to sexual potency and physical strength. The public needs a vast amount of counter-propaganda, but it also needs a positive approach and one that brings in all health workers but especially the doctors. Britain has slowly improved its control over new medicines offered to the medical profession, and has mitigated the worst abuses of the old 'patent medicines', but much needs to be done to establish a safe range of home medicaments and to make them available without false claims. The whole subject is intricate and expensive; and it may be that ultimately this part of the treatment of 'disease' will need to be taken out of the market-place, like scientific medicine.

Meantime health workers as a whole need to be brought into this part of the battle for health. There is too much tendency for those specializing in a narrow field to ignore or indeed not to know much about the wider fields of health and disease. Their training may give them no more insight into ways of health than the lay public has, and certainly no impulse to pass on what help they can. This is something they cannot be left to do without instruction, for we are all prone to folklore and superstitions, and there are more old wives' tales about health than about any other subject. It is true to a considerable extent that even those who accept the agreed teachings of scientific medicine will still retain much that has no connection with those teachings. In other words, health education cannot be a haphazard affair left to chance, but must be part of every health worker's curriculum.

While it would be ideal if every doctor and every health worker could play a full part in educating the public, it must be recognized that many lack the facility to talk and put over scientific knowledge in simpler language. There must, therefore, be a body of people who are professionally concerned with the subject and who are experts in telling the public about it. The Health Education Council has some responsibility for this but it does not handle all the material that is issued on health problems. It has always been said that it does not have enough money to do the best possible job and it is separate from the Department of Health. In a national health service it is vital that the public relations work should be done by the responsible department, and that health education should be seen as an important part of the central department's work. The present chairman of the Health Education Council, Baroness Birk, has made it clear that she and her colleagues are fully aware of the importance of their work. But it is too remote from the ordinary doctors and health workers to be able to mount a full-bodied programme even on the most obvious subjects. No one can be unaware of the claims for preservation of the teeth made by manufacturers of toothpaste. The efforts of the Health Education Council to put over the fully documented scientific claims for fluoridation of water supplies have had some success, but a measure of success such as the tooth-paste sellers would consider a failure.

It should be easy to organize education of the public in health. Everyone is interested in his or her own health, and the press, radio and television all find that health and medical subjects attract large audiences. Over the years all the mass media have featured the doctor, usually fictionally, but whenever possible, and whether in a favourable light or not, in true-story fashion. New advances, especially those like heart transplants with a dramatic element, are given full space and time. Science fiction features medical men in sequences that depict fantastic techniques not yet known to medical men. Children's programmes take up medical stories in a variety of ways. All this indicates that there is a public readiness to look at and listen to medical subjects, but no Western country seems to be using all the available techniques or putting the money into this important social need—education in the improvement and preservation of health.

Before we leave the subject it must be noted that the medical profession collectively has moved forward in this matter of educating the public on medical matters; not precisely on health education, but rather in assuming responsibility for advising the public. Fluoridation has already been mentioned, and is one subject on which the medical and dental professions have almost unanimously supported this way of assisting with the great problem of dental caries. More unanimously, and with greater vigour, the doctors, led by the Royal College of Physicians, have told the world exactly what the smoking of cigarettes can do to health. In one way, even more important than summarizing the evidence, which is largely statistical, and so has to be interpreted, the medical profession has taken its own advice and smoking among doctors has almost disappeared. Most medical bodies no longer permit smoking at their meetings. It is also significant in this connection that the Socialist Medical Association was the first medical body to come out against smoking, indicating that in this and other health matters political and medical views may coincide.

Health worker education must, however, be mainly in technical matters. Here we enter on a field bewildering in its diversity. But there is fairly general agreement that the health team must work together even if training and duties appear far apart. The Department of Health lists twenty-nine professional and technical workers and to this must be added trained nurses, enrolled nurses and midwives. Some of the groups could be subdivided still further. For example, laboratory technicians cover at least five quite distinct internal divisions, even if all students get the same basic training. If we stretch the definition into the managerial, clerical and craftsmen grades, there are many who require special training and whose duties are vital in a technical sense, such as sterilizer attendants, needle sharpeners and instrument curators.

This is not only a national problem, but one which WHO has recognized as needing a great deal of international agreement. In its 1968 study *Medical, Dental and Pharmaceutical Auxiliaries*, WHO lists the legislation that eighteen countries have already passed in efforts to regularize the training of auxiliaries. The lists of legislation may not be complete, but for South Africa there are given 38 Acts, orders and notices and for France 28. The UK has only 13 items in the list but this is because much of the necessary rules are embodied in one Act (1960), which set up registers for the professions supplementary to medicine. The medical and dental registers have long been the record of who is fully qualified to practise in Britain; now the same pattern of training, examination and registration has been set up for most of the auxiliary workers.

Some see in these arrangements a typical British compromise, for while employment in the NHS is conditional on specified training, much of which may be 'in service' training, the examining body is a voluntary organization, usually one established years ago by the auxiliary workers themselves. The additional factor is that under the 1960 Act each of the professional groups included now has an official board which has to satisfy itself that the training and examinations are of suitable standard; and these boards have certain disciplinary powers and can cancel a registration for proven misconduct in a professional sense.

This compromise, with its older example in the General Medical Council, which governs medical education and also has disciplinary powers, raises a very important question: to what extent should the Department of Health have a controlling influence over medical and health worker education? At present its influence is indirect, and this is praised because it gives the boards and the council independence and cushions them against political changes in government; yet there is always the danger that such bodies will become very rigid in their views and backward looking when the NHS needs forward-looking views. By the nature of things it is the elders of professions who are elected to controlling bodies, and it may be that the education of all health workers will have to be subject to much more departmental and ministerial supervision.

The definition of auxiliary professions raises many questions too detailed to be answered here as to the kind of salary and promotion ladder there should be in the NHS. The service needs a very simple scale that shows some similarity in the rewards to those whose degree of responsibility, size of department, age and experience are much alike, even if the jobs are vastly different. At present each group has separate agreements. It is probable that unless salaries can be seen to be sufficiently high for everyone there will be a continuous struggle for differentials in pay. One thing that needs to be considered is the possibility of movement, at least early in the career, from one profession to another, and above all from an auxiliary profession to medicine. There are always people who begin in one type of post and find it is not what they want, but cannot move into something they realize would suit them much better. In the Soviet Union it is said to be very easy, and the State makes appropriate grants for a health worker who after some training decides he, or more usually she, would like to qualify as a doctor. Clearly certain academic standards are necessary, but in a new integrated service it is to be hoped that flexibility not rigidity will be the keynote for the whole service.

The education of the doctor cannot escape, and has not escaped, the surge of changes in new universities and the greater surge due to social change. An integrated health service, the inauguration of the era of team-work rather than individual effort, the separation of private practice from the NHS and the development of full social responsibility among health workers, will all compel changes in medical education. Technological change will force the pace, for the computer is now an accepted tool in the health service; record linkage and record retrieval will speed up work and improve communication, and political developments will encourage rapid changes. The teaching hospital, once the ivory tower of the specialist busy with private practice, will take its place as a district hospital responsible for a unit of population as never before. The number of doctors and other health workers will continue to rise and recruitment will be from a wider range in society, so that social understanding will increase. The students themselves will demand changes in the way they are taught and they will learn faster than their predecessors by the use of the many modern visual and auditory teaching devices. The world need for more doctors and nurses will keep pressure on the authorities to change curricula, as well as methods, so that the need is more quickly met.

The present educational systems in most countries make much the same demand on medical students, but the one most successful in producing doctors has been the USSR. According to figures given by John Fry, the USSR produces 12.2 doctors per 100,000 of population, the US produces 3.75 and the UK 3.2 (the 1969 figure was, however, 3.8). There is a wide difference in the sex of doctors, 65 per cent in the USSR being women, 25 per cent in Britain and only 5 per cent in the US. The number of women students in Britain is rising and will increase further as medical schools attain an annual intake of 200, and new medical schools get into full production of graduates. It seems unlikely that either the UK or the USSR will shorten the medical training period, but the US, which has a longer training than the others, will probably cut out one year. Part of the argument about medical education concerns the very long training period, which with the time needed for specialist training postpones the time when a doctor can settle down and feel he is earning a proper living. On the other hand, the USSR requires medical graduates to do three years' service in a place or service ordered by the State; and America is seriously considering replacing the present 'draft' which puts young doctors into the armed forces with two years' service in rural areas. This is a familiar thought in medical circles which want to preserve private practice in the cities, but recognize that the rural areas need service. The older doctors, in developed and underdeveloped countries, think in terms of compelling young graduates to do two or three years in the wilderness while their elders make money in the cities. The same proposition has been put forward in the US and in India.

In Norway on the other hand there has been a system, said to go back 300 years and more, of making medical service in even the most remote areas attractive in terms of money, conditions of service, holidays and pensions. There are a few very remote areas in which it is difficult to get recruits but, Karl Evang says, 'there is generally no difficulty in obtaining qualified applicants for the jobs'. The doctors who take the posts, as we noted in an earlier chapter, are both public health doctors and physicians of primary care, and both elements of their work are paid for by a special scale. In Britain we have long had somewhat similar arrangements for the Highlands and Islands scheme in Scotland, but in general we have got better distribution of general practitioners by the negative pressure method of closing over-doctored areas and opening under-doctored areas to all who care to go there. Distribution is still not even in any section of health care but in an integrated service it can be improved. In a salaried service it should be simple to give financial incentives in areas which for a variety of reasons do not at present attract candidates. One big force in getting this done will be the formation of teams of doctors so that however isolated he may be by geography the individual physician will know and feel he is backed by the whole team.

A second factor will be the steady increase in the number of medical graduates produced in Britain. The Department of Health now has a manpower division which has the task of trying to match the training of all health workers against the possible number which will be needed in the future. In *Health Trends* (May 1971) Dr Kilgour, then in charge of this problem, wrote: 'In the foreseeable future, and not only in the UK, the demand for medical time is likely to exceed the doctors available to meet it, and in these terms there will be a shortage of doctors in the UK for many years to come'. Because of the twin traditions of British doctors going to the countries once under British control and doctors from old British territories coming to the UK for training, we have both an outflow and an inflow of medical men. Training doctors is a costly business but for many years Britain has taken more than it has given. Dr Kilgour's article gives a wealth of detail and shows clearly how much Britain depends in certain grades of hospital doctor on the men and women coming from Commonwealth countries. In

September 1970 overseas doctors formed 33.2 per cent of all the hospital staffs in England and Wales. It is particularly interesting, and indicates how good the basic training is in most countries today, that one-eighth of the consultants and one-fifth of senior registrars were born overseas. At one time the arrival of overseas doctors and their establishment in jobs was a very haphazard affair, but today a scheme of 'attachment' which gives the overseas graduate a period of clinical acclimatization is making both entry to Britain and progress in training much better. Many British graduates go abroad for periods of experience and it is now accepted that the average net loss, that is the minority who do not return, is about 300 a year. Many go to the US where the shortage is greater than it is in the UK. In Britain, 'our solution to our problem is to try to relate as fast as we can production of our own doctors to our own effective demand'. That is one laudable aim, but Dr Kilgour adds that we need not only an increase in total numbers but also better training, through 'providing better career counselling to the students and young doctors'. There is, of course, a limit to the numbers the medical schools can take, but there is room for expansion. In 1970, 2,873 doctors obtained first registrable medical qualifications. In the same year the Government announced that it intended to expand the medical school entry to 4,100 in the late 1970s.

No one will wish to interrupt the movement of medical graduates between countries, and as better arrangements for the care of tourists and visitors are made there will also be more movement among health workers. In an organized service like the NHS it will become increasingly important for service overseas to be recognized and encouraged, and it should therefore be by 'secondment', so that anyone working abroad has his rights in the NHS preserved. This already applies in some schemes. Teaching hospitals in the UK already exchange staffs with Indian and African hospitals, but this needs expansion and acceptance as a normal part of the career structure.

One point may cause difficulty, particularly in making new arrangements inside the Common Market: there is a wide divergence in the training and recognition of specialists. The NHS lists 34 specialties to which consultants are appointed: the USSR has 73. Many countries have very strict legislation on the subject, others leave the matter very open. There is a great contrast between the US definition—'By specialist is meant the man who claims to limit his work to his specialty', and the simple British NHS definition of a specialist as 'a medical officer appointed to the NHS for the purpose of practising a special branch of medicine with full responsibility for the treatment of patients' (*Medical Specialization*, WHO, 1958). In the course of time that definition has been clarified by the recognition within the NHS that a specialist will normally have a diploma from one of the Royal Colleges or another body which gives special training and holds special examinations. Since brilliance and genius may not fit into that pattern, however, the definition is not couched in legal terms but is left to an unwritten agreement within the service. At some point other nations may have to be persuaded that this is a good and accurate way of defining all specialists so that international movement can be made possible.

Specialization and the taking of examinations are part of the postgraduate education of every country. There are two aspects of this kind of further education, one directed to a special subject and examination, the other that continuous re-education of every doctor which the rapidity of modern advances makes imperative. This further education also has two facets, the formal education which consists of set courses within a specialty, and the less formal meetings of scientific bodies, medical associations and local groups. In the UK both aspects are today covered very fully. The formal part is largely controlled and organized by the British Postgraduate Medical Federation, which is a college of the University of London constituted by the federation of fifteen institutes of postgraduate training. It is concerned not only with university institutions but also with the hospital boards and with the appointment to posts in which the holder rotates between medical schools and a district general hospital. As more and more instruction for general practitioners is organized, the Federation joins in the organizing of refresher courses for general practitioners, courses recognized as official for various purposes by the Department of Health.

In British hospitals during the past fifteen years the idea of a hospital medical centre, originally fostered as an experiment at Kingston-upon-Thames by the King Edward's Hospital Fund for London, has spread and developed, and there are now over 200 such centres. Each hospital organizes its own meetings, designed for both consultants and general practitioners, and providing a common meeting ground for all the doctors of an area. The British Medical Association, which also arranges scientific and clinical meetings, may use the same premises; and set courses may also be organized locally or regionally. Attendance at such meetings is one of the factors in the consideration of general practitioners for seniority payments. In such medical centres the concept of the district medical team, closely knit but actively engaged in the necessary exchange of views and new ideas, is bringing nearer to full realization the co-operation that will be essential to an integrated service.

Postgraduate education is also a feature of international co-operation, and ranges from the annual or occasional conferences of people drawn from many countries but practising the same specialty to the organizing of training of individual doctors from many countries. There are now many fellowships in medical subjects which involve foreign experience, and many charitable foundations which appoint foreign doctors to posts abroad. The British Postgraduate Medical Federation has four officers concerned entirely with the placing and exchange of postgraduate students from all over the world. The British Council sends British specialists to lecture at medical schools in many countries with some emphasis on places where English is used in training. This co-operation, fortunately and as a good omen for the future, ignores boundaries, and the doctors of the US and the USSR, and indeed of the world, are becoming increasingly accustomed to meeting at international gatherings on many subjects.

Behind all this, and the basic need for any system of health care, are the undergraduate medical schools, each with its hospital or group of hospitals in which the clinical teaching is mainly done. It is paradoxical, and probably has been over the centuries, that most UK medical schools have a very long history but all are in an almost continuous state of change and often of debate. Medicine itself requires change, and everyone who has spent a lifetime in medical service can look back over a time of continuous change not only in the body of knowledge taught but in all the accompanying technology. That will go on as long as medicine is growing and developing; today there are also a whole host of changes arising on the one hand from the need to organize medical care on a new basis, and on the other because students are no longer content to receive their training as if medicine was a dogma, but want to influence both the methods of teaching and the content of what is taught. Here anyone trying to look ahead to the changes which will have to be made in a fully integrated service in a society which is itself changing and is liable also to violent change, can probably do no more than plead for flexibility. The cherished routine of examinations which in the past produced our medical graduates is now as seriously questioned as any other item in training. The content of the curriculum is based on the past and has little in it that looks forward. Above all it has not moved fast enough to recognize that while Britain retains the general practitioner as the primary care physician, and while the training of specialists is recognized to be, rightly, a lengthy process, no adjustments have been made to the routes by which these two differing groups of doctors have to reach maturity.

In thinking about this one should remember, as Dr Ian R. McWhinney did in *The Lancet* (14 January 1967), that 'an accident of history has given us a referral system between primary physicians and specialists which is ideally suited to the delivery of medical care'. (Dr McWhinney thought that 'countries who are not so fortunate may well have to invent a system similar to our own'). He thought that it was tragic that this being so our doctors 'are taught in a sphere utterly remote from primary care and by physicians who have had little experience of it'. The changes are however even more profound than is suggested by that adherence to the teaching hospital. Not only has the whole epidemiology of what the primary care doctor has to deal with altered; he now needs many more 'behavioural and sociological insights in diagnosis and treatment', which are vastly different from those needed by the specialist. Dr McWhinney thought that medical education had suffered very often in the past from the failure of teachers in medical schools to recognize the changes that were taking place within the practice of medicine, and especially in fields outside the hospitals. New special subjects were not included in orthodox teaching: 'The same thing is happening now with primary medicine. At a time when all the specialist disciplines are at last being drawn together, medical schools still do not see it as their job to provide primary care, to do research into its problems, or to teach it to undergraduates and postgraduates'.

The position has in fact improved since those words were written. Professors in General Practice have appeared on the scene; Guy's Hospital in London has developed and become very involved in the Thamesmead project in which its Department of Community Medicine will be doing the kind of provision and research that is needed. The teaching hospitals have been told that they must regard themselves as district hospitals, the New Charing Cross Hospital at its new premises in Fulham being an example. It cannot fail to be involved in the community at its new site in a working-class area of high population density, but will be more effectively involved when all its consultants are out of private practice and find new links, new interests, even new excitements in a closely knit community.

The technicalities of what should now be taught to students have to be worked out by educationalists, but one thing must be quite clear. However the curriculum is altered, and however the effort to teach the basic principles and knowledge of medical science is made, not only must all students be taught about the social implications of the NHS: they must at some point be given experience of primary care. No matter what specialty a doctor means to follow, including primary care, the unity of the health team, not its present divided nature, must be among the things demonstrated. When it was decided that all medical graduates must do one year in the hospitals before registration, many thought that in addition to or as part of that year every graduate should do six months at a health centre. The idea failed because there were no health centres. Now we can go back to it, as health centres and group practices would make it quite feasible to give every graduate a real insight into the base on which the delivery of British health care is built.

There are many subsidiary problems to be settled. With the present length of study before graduation, the pre-registration year, the need for primary care experience and the tradition of doing at least one extra hospital year, the average doctor is at least twenty-five years of age before he is ready to settle down either to health centre practice or to the long road to consultancy. Society has to recognize that marriage and family are now thought desirable at a much earlier age than formerly, and if we are to select and put through this long training over 4,000 students a year, grants and living accommodation for students, and incomes and living conditions for young doctors, all need to be improved. It is already quite a costly business to train a doctor. It will cost the future society much more, and this is another reason why, having used the nation's resources for training, the qualified doctor should give the whole of his time to the country's service. It has been suggested that students should regard their grants as loans to be repaid in money; but as we advance to a more ethical society a return as service is more important than a return in cash.

In addition to a better promotional structure the NHS requires a system that offers fairly straightforward movement within its framework. At present, each young doctor has to seek his own appointments, and may find the task of shopping around, especially if he has married and started a family, quite a drain on his energy. Slowly efforts have been made to give better counselling to students and young doctors so that they find the field that best suits their skills; and those who have started to specialize are greatly assisted by rotating schemes for hospital registrars and senior registrars. Young doctors have in recent years organized to get better conditions, better incomes and better training, and if the service is to go on advancing these demands must be met. One essential is the need for a definition of the roles of specialists and consultants. In

NHS documents the terms have been used as if they were synonymous, or as if it is necessary to use them together to make their separate status and duties clear. In fact the title of specialist needs to be moved down the age and training scale to a point where young doctors have made a personal decision to specialize and have been accepted in a training post. The registrar by his second year at that grade is already a specialist in this sense, and is certainly so when he is appointed Senior Registrar. After one year in such a post, when he has to be certified by his immediate seniors as suitable for further training and likely to achieve higher appointments, he is doing full specialist work as a member of the team, and often taking a very high degree of responsibility. He is also taking examinations in his special subject. There comes a point however when promotion and salary increases cease, and some men and women have a long period of waiting before they become consultants and start on the next series of annual increments.

At the other end of the scale, 3,300 consultants are being paid 'merit awards', producing a further disparity, for these extra payments do not represent extra hard work, extra hours of work or additional administrative duties. To some extent they are little more than an additional increment, for in 1969, 25 rewards of £1,000 a year were given to people under 40 years of age, and of the 338 rewards 159, almost half, were given to consultants under the age of 48. Since no one knows who these 159 meritorious ones were, or what their merit was, the additional salary given at that age represents nearly £5 million added to the earnings of this group of consultants before their retirement at 65.

The annual cost of merit awards is now over £9 million, and the method of award a very poor way of deciding where such a large sum of money should go. However well the committee which makes the awards does it – and no one questions that they try to do what their terms of reference dictate – the money could be much better applied in a new and longer incremental scale for specialists. This could absorb all the C (£1,200) and B (£2,820) awards into the salary, so that the man now known as Senior Registrar would be, simply, a specialist, and would have a chance of climbing a bit further before coming to the top of his scale. Consultants would then become what the title says, not only those who have specialized, who can do a first-class job in their subject even if they show no innovative brilliance, but those who have more to give than mere technical skill, and who are consulted by their colleagues. The money now paid in A (£4,800) and A plus (£6,330) awards should then be attached to posts advertised as carrying special duties, and demanding special skills. These would make a base for the consultants' ladder, which should overlap and exceed in years that of the specialists. This is not to suggest a system of chiefs and assistants, but a change of nomenclature within the team, recognizing that the team would usually consist of members with different degrees of the skill in the work with which each team was concerned. It would also get rid of the 'secrecy' of merit awards, which had its origin, like so many other things, in the profession's attempt to retain private practice. Doctors do not like to face competition, and it was felt that the public announcement that Dr A. had a merit award while Dr B. did not would lead to all private patients going to one man. In a salaried service with salary scales publicly advertised this competition would vanish and be replaced by a recognition of merit arising from the job a man was doing, and not from some theoretical merit in his past history.

Education in all the senses we have discussed is very obviously of social importance, and requires changes in views and changes in institutions. To meet the challenge of the next twenty years our students should be getting instruction in the medicine of AD 2,000. Since few teachers have that kind of vision all we can do is to try to build flexibility into curriculum and teaching, instil an attitude of attention to the ever-changing social environment, and provide enough continuing education to justify our hope that at very least we are up to date. But all these necessary changes require some kind of guidelines, new decisions and new initiatives: a blueprint for a new NHS.

The Blueprint

Chapter 18

The Health Centre Team

Plans, blueprints, Green Papers and White Papers, together with books and pamphlets on the next stage of development in Britain's National Health Service crowd the desks of students, university professors and administrators. They are the direct descendants of the first declarations in favour of an organized health service made at the turn of the century. For Dr Benjamin Moore, writing *The Dawn of the Health Age* in 1910, the needs could be simply expressed.

> Just now there is a great and general awakening of the public mind, voiced by the thoughts and actions of millions of the best of the inhabitants of the country, towards a real scientific and continued endeavour to deal with the problems of poverty and disease in a way that means eradication from the race and not merely amelioration of the lot of the individual.

To Professor Peter Townsend in *Labour and Inequality* sixty years later there is need for a great programme of social planning, which will, however, make no sense if it is confined to the public health, welfare, education, housing and social security services, and does not also include industrial welfare services and the social aspects of income tax, environmental and manpower policies. The language has changed but the aspiration is the same: to eradicate poverty and disease from the community and to do it by planned means. Roy Jenkins, MP, speaking on 11 March 1972, made the same point: 'The next Labour Government can be content with nothing less than the elimination of poverty as a social problem. Britain already has sufficient resources to remove the abuses of remaining poverty'. Democracy is often slow-moving, and it took thirty-five years from the date of Moore's first writings to put on the statute book the health service he wanted and first helped to devise—a slow process. In the words of Almont Lindsey (*Socialized Medicine*): 'The National Health Service, then, was not hastily foisted upon the nation by a Labour Government in the excitement of the post-war years. It was the evolutionary result of many years of planning and it had the broadest sort of bipartisan support'.

Today everyone is agreed on two points. First, as Sir Keith Joseph has said, 'we have a potentially superb National Health Service'. Secondly, to achieve the whole potential, changes must be made. The tripartite administration must be ended and one integrated service planned that will carry the service over the next twenty-five years as the first plan has done over the last quarter of a century. Lindsey said of that plan that it was 'a compromise among the realities of the past, the imperatives of the present and the hopes of the future'. Aneurin Bevan, writing in 1952 (*In Place of Fear*), described how first hygiene and later active prevention had improved the health of Western countries; no one had expected those advances to be achieved other than by public action and with public money. Now, he said, the same story

> 'is being unfolded in the field of curative medicine. Here individual and collective action are joined in a series of dramatic battles. The collective principle asserts that the resources of medical skill and the apparatus of healing shall be placed at the disposal of the patient, without charge, when he or she needs them; that medical treatment and care should be a communal responsibility; that they should be made available to rich and poor alike in accordance with medical need and by no other criteria. It claims that financial anxiety in time of sickness is a serious hindrance to recovery, apart from its unnecessary cruelty. It insists that no society can legitimately call itself civilised if a sick person is denied medical aid because of lack of means.

All of that, one can assume, is now part of the British way of life, and what we need for the future is a better and fuller realization of these ideals.

Before starting on a detailed examination of that new plan, however, we have to look at AD 2,000 and consider in the widest terms what the position of the human race is likely to be; and some formidable problems stand in the way of any clear view. The most pessimistic forecast, especially among the group who call themselves ecologists, is that by that date the world population will have grown so rapidly that it will, on the one hand, be unable to provide food for all, and on the other will be using up the surface of the earth and all the materials available within that part of the surface that man can and does exploit: he will have wasted his total inheritance. The population explosion is a world phenomenon. India needs to build a city the size of Birmingham every month to house her new people;

the world needs a new Plymouth every day with all the schools, hospitals, factories and so on that such a city must have. The motor-car threatens to cover the surface so thickly that while transport becomes more and more difficult, the whole of the oil that can still be pumped from the crust of the globe will be used up and converted into atmospheric pollution. By AD 2,000 we will have spent vast amounts of the world's wealth and energy on space exploration without finding another place which the human species could exploit for its own survival. We will not have learned that violence and war should have no part in the life of such a small world, and the waste of men and money on so-called defensive measures will still not have been replaced by world government. In the health field we will not have solved the problems of the great killers – heart and blood-vessel diseases, cancer in all its forms – or lessened man's addiction to poisonous substances. The under-developed areas of the world will still have impossibly low per capita incomes, and the most primitive parts of the human race, the aboriginal people of great areas of South America, for example, will have been destroyed to make room for their technologically skilled brothers from other countries. There will be more human beings who could be usefully employed making with their hands things they need, and doing jobs like preparing sterile materials for the medical service and improving the homes of the people; but present attempts to automate all that work succeeds only in throwing people out of work (and so into poverty and ill health), and converts more and more energy into chemical and radio-active pollutants. The change necessary to prevent this is both political and ethical. Professor Barry Commoner declared in *The Observer* (12 March 1972) that the alternatives lie outside technology: 'Our use of power is extraordinarily wasteful because it is governed mainly by the profit motive. The whole issue of limits on resources can be resolved only by modifying the social system'. He declared himself an optimist but his forebodings were deeply pessimistic.

In such a world the health services would still not be getting enough money to save and succour not only the sick, but also the increasing millions of elderly living some kind of medicated life, Shakespearian in some senses if not completely 'without everything'. The optimists can deny much of this picture, but not the population increase; and are compelled to admit that unless we could have a universal halt on childbearing for something like a decade, millions more will have to be fed every year. It is possible that the more advanced countries will reduce their birth rates and that their numbers may soon cease to increase, but the problem remains and will go on growing in most underdeveloped areas. In such areas medical science, no matter how few doctors they have, is improving conditions, and as the infections come under control more children survive and the population increases. Expectation of life may rise ahead of any improved industrialization or even cultivation, and the pressure on food will not greatly slacken although the so-called 'green revolution' has pushed up the output of home-grown foods from improved seeds and better fertilisers. The optimists among scientists believe enough can be produced to feed the expected population of AD 2,000, even if the production has to include artificially produced protein from yeasts and bacteria. Man's skill and ingenuity will certainly overcome some of the problems, but every solution seems to have inherent new difficulties. Atomic energy may contribute more and more to the world's usable power but leave a problem of how to get rid of radio-active wastes which could harm the whole race if not effectively dealt with outside the earth's atmosphere.

While we wait to see who is right the world will go on producing goods, manufacturing more motor-cars and aeroplanes and building more and more sky-scraper collections of glass, steel and concrete boxes. If this is done within an unaltered form of ruthless capitalism the results can be disastrous even to those moving into the twenty-first century. If the whole world is to move into a new political, economic and ethical system the rate of change has to be revolutionary, and the degree of change has to be widespread. If poverty, for example, persists, diseases related to malnutrition and crowded and insanitary conditions will remain. The health services of most countries will still be orientated to the cure of disease, while the vision of a service designed to serve the healthy and improve the health of nations will be no more than a vision.

History, we may say, suggests this is not the most likely way things will go. When in 1908 the minority report on the Poor Law postulated a healthy nation served by a national medical service, the condition of the working class was only just beginning to move from the description Engels had written in the middle of the nineteenth century—'The pattern in which wage incomes before taxation are distributed has remained unchanged since 1886' (Jenkins). Britain has not rid itself of inequality, but it has increased the total wealth of the nation and softened the pressures of poverty even while some ten million people are still below the modestly computed line which guides a great deal of thinking on the subject. If we do no more than add together the unemployed, the physically and mentally disabled, the elderly, and their families, the amount of poverty in our society becomes very obvious. Such relief as they get mainly comes from their own money; from the insurance contributions they paid every week when they were working and from any savings they have. They are the people who are running the greatest risk of ill health, and without the NHS disease would be added to their poverty. But people do own more that they once did, and fewer live under conditions of desperate hardship even if a million homes still do not have a bathroom. We must assume that in the last quarter of this century organised labour will go on forcing the industrial system to pay better wages, and will force governments to achieve some redistribution of wealth so that medicine and medical men will be spared having to deal with too much poverty-induced disease. The social wage in Britain stands high compared with many countries, and it is in social welfare and in health care that we must expect a continuing transfer of wealth from the rich to the poor. It is therefore against a background which is not too desolate, and not without hope, and with the prospect of increasing national wealth, that we now look at health in the next two decades.

The principles of the NHS must remain unaltered, and as we have indicated in every field we have discussed, the one that has to be the focus of our attention is that of comprehensiveness. No one has seriously suggested that the service should be other than universally available, and it is therefore a comprehensive service for the whole nation and for those of Britain's visitors who require help that we have to plan. None of the three documents already issued on the subject, two Green Papers by Labour Secretaries of State and a 'Consultative Document' produced by their successor, Sir Keith Joseph, have offered a plan that has had more than half-hearted support from a minority; and time need not be spent looking at them further. While this book is in the printer's hands a Government White Paper may appear, based on Sir Keith Joseph's document and some exceedingly curious documents that have been sent round interested bodies for comment before the final draft appears. More than any previous documents these are exceedingly theoretical, draw nothing from past experience, and indicate nothing that would not be a mere passing phase. The Health Service at this moment has schemes for the nursing profession (Salmon), for medical administration (Cogwheel), and plans to make changes arising from the attempted reorganisation of social service. None of these seem likely to last in their present form, and certainly not if in the fairly near future there is a more radical government. Cogwheel was and is a most peculiar attempt to substitute a committee form of medical administration for a really responsible medical administrator. Its purpose, progress and failure are described in the annual report from the Chief Medical Officer, *On the State of the Public Health* (1970). 'Effective medical organization is essential to achieve high standards of patient care and at the same time the maximum use of limited resources'. The Cogwheel plan was an attempt to provide that effective medical organization, but 'the advantages of a Cogwheel system in seeking to achieve these objectives has yet to be fully validated'. It appears that only 138 out of 327 places (42 per cent) which should have put Cogwheel into operation have even made a start (May 1970). There were many places in the hospital service where the medical administrator and his clinical colleagues had established a good way of working and mutual co-operation, and would have made a better plan than Cogwheel. We return to it later but meantime have tried to indicate that none of the existing official proposals appear to fulfil any of the needs of a truly comprehensive democratic system.

If we start with the citizen and consider his or her needs individually and collectively we can then go to elaborate the changes needed, if any, in the delivery of care, and in administration, where the changes needed are many. The citizen in Britain has already got a good deal of what he needs, but he needs better techniques of delivery and a wider scope. It is still necessary to begin with diagnosis and treatment, and indeed there is no valid reason why they should not always have maximum priority. It is agreed that prevention is better than allowing a preventable disease to happen; but disease, however seemingly trivial, should never be neglected, for terminal illness begins very often with minor symptoms. But there is also the point that if a doctor, or other health worker, allows himself to think of symptoms as trivial, examinations as routine, and continuity unimportant, his own standards and judgements will rapidly deteriorate.

In diagnosis and treatment, then, we still need an organization of health workers of primary contact. The correct descriptive term for these health workers will be health centre workers, the doctor of primary contact will be a health centre physician. We would prefer the inclusion in his terms of reference of much that is called community medicine, and deprecate the tendency to speak loosely of a community physician without definition. Just as we want no boundaries between patient and any necessary service, we would prefer no boundary between any qualified physician and any part of the community he serves, and the invention of a so far undefined 'community physician' to replace the former Medical Officer of Health implies a misunderstanding of what the health centre team will have to do.

We have used the term 'health worker of first contact' because the moment our family doctors change to health centre team-work the questions of who sees every patient first in an illness, who joins in domiciliary care, and who initiates health education, all take on new meanings. It is, of course, essential to this move that the general practitioners of medicine and nursing are salaried officers of the new integrated services, and that any of either profession who wish to continue private practice will do so, as some already do, outside the NHS. The family doctor in the past ten years has reached a position in which so much of his NHS income takes the form of basic salary and regular payments that the move to a proper salary scale will be much less difficult than the profession thought at one time.

In discussing teams of health workers we can look more closely at some points in general practice which are slowly evolving. First there is the question of whether every first contact must be made by a qualified doctor, or whether the nurse, who has been trained and has experience in domiciliary care, can help the doctor and the patient by making some primary visits in the course of her home visiting. Secondly, we have to consider how real emergencies are to be dealt with and by whom. In our present divided service, accidents in the street and in many work places are the job of the emergency ambulance service; urgencies in the home are still the province of the GP. This leads, inevitably, to many cases where the GP is not available, is out on his round or has some other duty. Health centres will alter this to a considerable extent for, especially in centres with six or more doctors, there can be a rota which ensures that there is always one on emergency duty, including nights. Clearly the experienced nurse will join in these emergency calls, and at the health centres themselves she may have to take charge of emergency cases brought there. Will she have the clear duty, in the absence of a GP, to call whichever is necessary of the emergency services, accident, heart rescue teams, midwifery flying squad? The term nurse will in the next twenty years collect a great variety of meanings and the people involved, male and female, will have a great variety of duties.

The duties of the GP will be equally varied. Figure 18.1 attempts to set out how many they are and what interconnections must exist. It shows better than words why the GP of the future must be a specialist in this particular type of medicine and why he will need re-educating and refreshing during his whole professional life. We are postulating only one physician of primary care, but others have looked at this list of responsibilities and suggested it would be better to have more than one, for example general practitioner

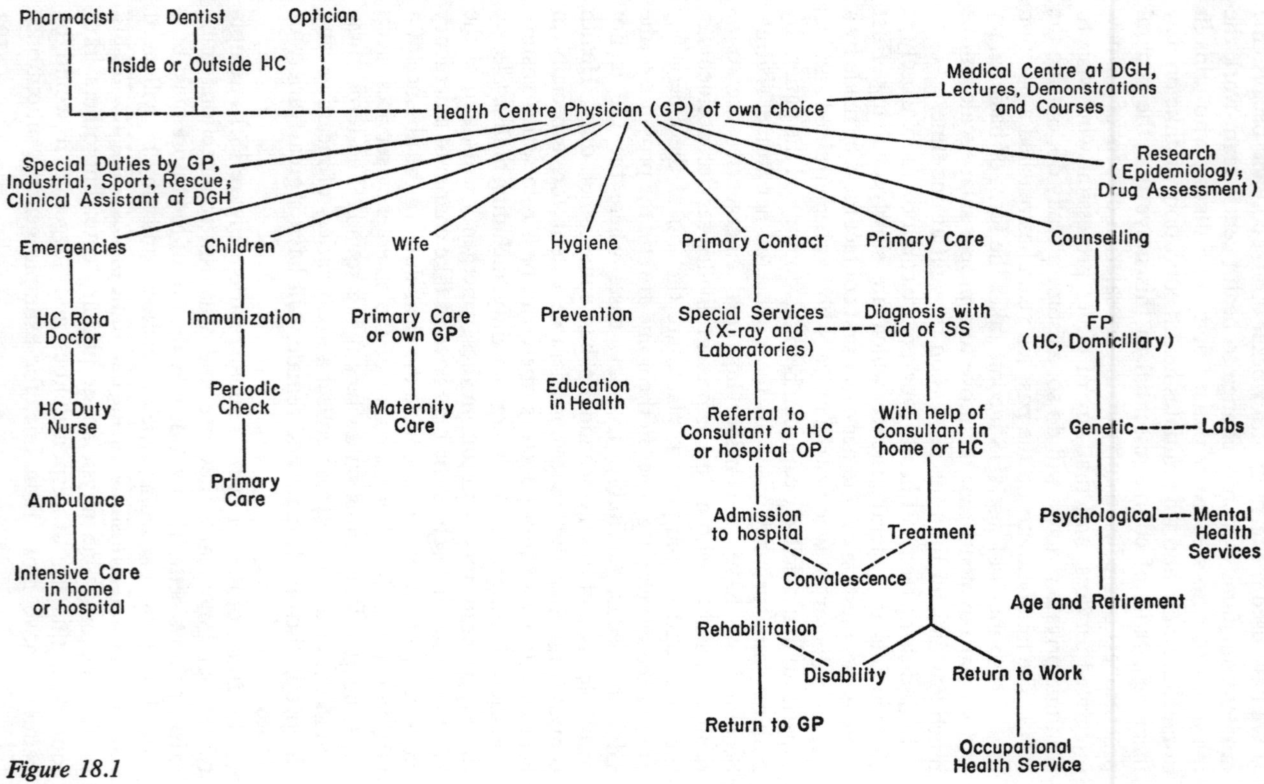

Pharmacist
Dentist
Optician
Inside or Outside HC
Health Centre Physician (GP) of own choice
Medical Centre at DGH, Lectures, Demonstrations and Courses
Special Duties by GP, Industrial, Sport, Rescue; Clinical Assistant at DGH
Research (Epidemiology; Drug Assessment)
Emergencies
HC Rota Doctor
HC Duty Nurse
Ambulance
Intensive Care in home or hospital
Children
Immunization
Periodic Check
Primary Care
Wife
Primary Care or own GP
Maternity Care
Hygiene
Prevention
Education in Health
Primary Contact
Special Services (X-ray and Laboratories)
Referral to Consultant at HC or hospital OP
Admission to hospital
Convalescence
Rehabilitation
Disability
Return to GP
Primary Care
Diagnosis with aid of SS
With help of Consultant in home or HC
Treatment
Return to Work
Occupational Health Service
Counselling
FP (HC, Domiciliary)
Genetic
Labs
Psychological
Mental Health Services
Age and Retirement

Figure 18.1

paediatricians, geriatricians or obstetricians. Every family doctor in Britain today may avoid obstetrics but not the other two, which indeed make up a large part of his work. Experiences in other countries do not suggest that we need a corps of doctors of first contact. The separation of children's doctors has been most successfully tried in the USSR, and most unsuccessfully developed in the USA. In the latter the primary care of children under private practice conditions has led to a sub-specialty of general practitioner-paediatrician, but it is expensive and incomplete and wasteful of manpower. In the USSR, however, the young medical student has to make an early decision to be a doctor either of children or of adults. If he decides on the care of the child, his education then excludes adult medicine and he is trained in the care of children both individually and collectively. This has certainly produced healthy children and a widely spread service, but there are many reasons why it is not favoured elsewhere. It is quite true that there are some diseases peculiar to childhood and some symptoms that are different in the young, but on the whole the division, like the age fixed for adulthood, is artificial. Above all it prevents the development of family doctors who look after the whole family and take into account the total environment. The familiar family doctor can very often handle children who know him better than the stranger, however experienced. The work involved in looking after children is today very much lighter than it was in the days of epidemics. The GP who has an average patient list of around 2,500 will have between 500 and 700 children in his care, but today he will have assistance from health visitors and nurses attached to him or his group. Many GPs run special services for their children.

Nor does there seem any way in which a separate group of geriatricians could work in health centres and homes quite separate from hospital beds and all the associated therapies, physical, recreational and occupational, which are now available. The family doctor will usually have known his ageing patients for a long time, and knows what treatments they have had. What he needs is a very full service from consultant geriatricians who have, above all, day hospital places at their disposal. This is one field in which the home nurse working with her day hospital colleagues will have an increasing part to play; and the day hospital nurses should not be confined to their institutions, for they may have a part to play in a better day bed service.

Obstetrics may benefit greatly from an integrated service. Under the NHS the pregnant woman has certainly had a choice, for all three sections of the service have provided a part or the whole of maternity care. This was in fact one of the clearest examples of the inherent errors in a tripartite service, for although almost all women got excellent care at every stage of the pregnancy they did not get it necessarily from one doctor or one source. While the number of births taking place in hospital has steadily increased to nearly 80 per cent the midwife, in both hospital and the home, has delivered most of the babies with the doctor, the GP or the consultant obstetrician and his staff being called upon for abnormalities and emergencies. We need not go into all the present complications of antenatal care given by GPs, by the domiciliary midwives and by hospital clinics, for they should all be amalgamated in an integrated service. The GP will therefore continue to play a part but it would seem likely, as fewer births take place at home, that within a health centre group one or two of the doctors, with the midwives, would take over the whole of the maternal care and midwifery for the whole group. (This kind of division of activities and specialisation within a group of health centre doctors was always envisaged as likely and desirable.)

The health centre physician in Britain and largely in Europe will continue to be in charge of primary care for individuals of both sexes – the physician may of course be of either sex and any age – and as his numbers increase yearly (by 230 in 1971) the average list will drop to a figure where the many items in Figure 18.1 will be well within his scope. By 1980 it may be possible to make the present average 2,500 the maximum, and the average well below that figure. In addition his work will be better organized, and as the recent report on group practice declared this is the best way of providing a higher standard of care. The well-organized health centre, at which all but emergency cases are seen by appointment, adequate reception and secretarial staff, nurses and health visitors working with their own team of doctors and the visits of such technical and medical specialists as are found necessary, will all make for a better way of life for the doctor and a better service for the sick. With more time to spare the health centre doctor will be able to give more time to the psychosomatic illnesses, and time to health education. Such preventive methods as we now have will be part of the daily routine of every health centre. The health centre doctor will widen his horizon. Research, especially into the epidemiology of disease, the effects of environment on health and the testing of new medicaments in the field (after their full laboratory checking), will not only add to the doctor's interests, but prove of great value to the service. One of the most valuable developments in the past ten or fifteen years has been the amount of research done by GPs, partly fostered by the Royal College of General Practitioners, and by special units such as the

General Practice Research Unit at Guy's Hospital in London. There, in connection with the Thamesmead community health project, so much research is found to be possible that a computer unit is in operation there to handle and store the data.

A glance at Figure 18.1 will show why it is impossible to continue with the present arrangement, under which the GP is a contractor of medical care, and why he must become the full-time salaried leader of the health centre team of salaried officers. He is now going to work in premises provided by the nation, a capital investment of up to £100 million by the time the whole country is so served, a capital outlay doctors could not meet and should not be expected to meet. The NHS took general practice out of the market-place when the buying and selling of practices was prohibited and compensation agreed; and it is impossible to go on to the next stage of advance if health centres, built by the taxpayer, are to be used for private profit by calling the GP a contractor and not an employee. The fears doctors once had were unjustified and have been shown to be so by the complete clinical freedom, and the large measure of control, which the salaried consultants of the hospital service have retained. Indeed the experience of British consultants matches that of their colleagues in Denmark and Norway that only in a salaried position can a specialist give of his very best to all the sick. The GPs will now have to follow and will no doubt fight for full recognition of the fact that the specialty of health centre physician is of equal standing with all other specialties.

There is one further question that is often debated and must be dealt with in any reorganization: the relation of the health centre doctor to the hospitals of his area, and whether he should, always and automatically, have duties, or some would say rights, in the hospital service. There is no published evidence that any large proportion of family doctors wish to be hospital specialists also: but it cannot be surprising, in view of the historical relationship of GPs to the old voluntary hospitals in Britain, which until forty years ago they largely staffed, that some want the opportunity of treating some of their patients in hospital beds. Like so many questions in the NHS this one has been bedevilled by the contractor status of the GP and by the use of NHS beds for private practice. Once the family doctor, like his hospital colleague, is a salaried officer, and the district team concept has been clarified and accepted, the position will be very different. Then it should be possible for each district health committee to look at its resources, and assess which hospitals can in fact be staffed by GPs, or in which hospitals GPs can look after their own cases when the latter do not require continuing consultant care.

Provided the health centre doctor's list of patients leaves him with the time, then those GPs who want to treat their own cases in an available smaller hospital should be able to do so. Nowhere in the original discussions on hospital planning was it ever considered that small hospitals would be abolished. But we have not in the past sufficiently educated either the doctors or the people about what we want hospitals to do to have achieved a rational plan. Some very small, some very old hospitals are positively dangerous if used for surgery and other specialties; hospitals where a GP can attend to such of his patients who need expert nursing but not the specialist, and where the GP confines himself to 'things within his own competence,' may have a place in planned service. Much depends on the staff available in any area and the distances to be covered. Where the district general hospital is more than a few miles away, there is a strong case to be made for small hospitals as 'return stations', to which post-operation and semi-convalescent cases might be sent for a few days extra but less expensive hospital care. Day surgery has proved that cases operated on for minor surgical conditions can be sent home to be nursed by the district nurse under the GP. What is needed is flexibility in planning coupled with completely competition-free team work.

Mention of day surgery, day hospitals and return stations in a health centre system indicates how correct the first pioneers were in proposing a service that must not be over-centralised, and in which the patient is to be taken to the service or vice versa, whichever is better. Another thing which needs to be both flexible and freely available is transport for the sick. Home visiting is an essential feature of the primary care system we are discussing, but there will always be cases that need not be confined to bed, but need transport to their health centre. Experiments in Scotland, Wales and London have already shown that many patients benefit from such a system, although not all liked it, and some doctors found they lost more time waiting for delayed patients than they would have spent in visiting them; and the cost was very high. It is a subject that must be studied on the spot, for geography is important and is another reason why the basic health service unit must not be too large. Transport of patients from remote areas to main hospitals may, even in a country of Britain's size, necessitate the use of air transport. The hospitals of the future will almost certainly use helicopters for the movement of patients to central units for special types of care—burns and brain surgery are two that have already had this kind of service.

The health centre physician requires the help not only of those who may act under his instruction, but from specialists of all kinds. There should be no conflict over whether all consultants should still be seen at their hospital consultative clinics, or should visit the health centres in their area. This should be a matter for local decision, depending on the size of the health centre and therefore the number of cases a consultant might expect to see at a session, and of course the distances involved and the availability of public transport. It may be simpler for one consultant to drive himself to a distant centre than for ten or twenty cases to get to the district hospital. What is important is that the hospital consultants should be mobile, ready to see patients if convenient at the health centre, but also to meet their colleagues in domiciliary consultation. One consultant service, clinical pathology, is often spoken of as if every health centre would have its own laboratory; some speak of having a technician there as well. The Group Laboratory system was started, and has persisted and grown, because in this field concentration of work is easy, is more accurate when done in numbers (especially with the automatic machines of today and the better ones that may be devised tomorrow), and enables the consultant pathologists to advise on many more cases. It is also more economic in terms of scarce qualified technicians. But here again flexibility and local planning are essential, and a variety of systems may work so long as every health centre doctor gets the service he needs.

That applies also to X-rays, and there is very little to be said for spreading small and inefficient (but expensive) equipment at many points where it may be badly used. The place for X-rays is a hospital large enough to merit first-class equipment and staff. Laboratories and X-ray raise the question of screening populations for hidden defects or doing multiphasic screening of whole populations in the expectation of detecting early disease. There is a great deal of misunderstanding of what can be done in this field, how much early disease can be detected, proved and treated, and at what price. The idea that everyone should annually have a complete set of blood tests done (twelve or more), an X-ray of the chest, in the case of women a cervical smear, and so on, is most commonly held in the private sector of medicine in which it produces very high incomes for those who do it. The British attitude is much more cautious. If priorities are considered and national spending on health is limited, it is much more important that the family doctor faced with a query should be able to turn to the laboratory and all his consultant colleagues and get everything done without question, and without charge. In so far as screening is done, and it will undoubtedly increase, it should be done for specific purposes for which accurate tests are available, and for which immediate treatment is freely available. It is no use doing many blood chemical tests just because we have machines that do them all on one sample of blood, if we cannot take action on all the results. It must always be remembered that no matter how good our machines are, on average they have an in-built error or at least variation which may be greater than the range of abnormality for which we are searching. Working with an instrument with a 5 per cent error is not much value if the disease tested for occurs in only 1 per cent of the population. It must be said, however, that if in this decade we have statistical evidence that multiphasic screening is of value then our health centres will be ideal places for the collection of samples and the collation of results.

One question that health centres and salaried doctors will inevitably raise is that of hours of work. For most health workers, in hospitals and clinics, hours are part of negotiated terms of service, and in many grades overtime or even bonus payments are the rule. The doctor has by the nature of his work been less prone to ask for fixed hours, and even those full-time officers in departments which close at a specific hour know that when on call for emergency there is no timetable. The GP has never had hours worked out because as a contractor he is legally responsible for all his list patients every minute the year long. In practice he makes arrangements with colleagues for leave and recreation; in groups and health centres he makes internal arrangements which satisfy the law but allow each doctor time off; or he may use one of the emergency services that have sprung up to meet this need. The concept of health centres visualizes a group of doctors who cover all their collective patients every minute of every day, but who organize their work as efficiently as they can. Part of that efficiency is that everyone gets his quota of time off—not only for recreation but for attending meetings and so on. The yardstick will almost certainly be the number of doctors per so many thousand citizens, based on national and regional averages, and a great deal of liberty will be left to the doctors in the organization of their working time. But once again local democracy will have a great deal to say if the service falls below what is expected. In passing it may be noted that in the hospitals an exact working day has never been laid down, the consultants working to a 'notional half-day' which is used in a calculation as to how many sessions are needed to cover a certain number of beds and consultative clinics, and in the case of surgeons how many hours must be spent in operating theatres.

In writing of the family doctor's relation with the hospital we have already discussed one item shown in Figure 18.1, visits to the medical centre for lectures, demonstrations and courses. This is something in which there may be big developments during the next few years. Medical centres, libraries and museums are all necessary in a health service and must be included in any new hospitals being built. In addition the visits of consultants to a health centre must always have in them an element of re-education for all the staff with whom the consultant comes in contact. If he is also keen on health education for the public then his visits to the centres can be used in that way. Among the consultants who may organize their work so as to include sessions at health centres are all those concerned with mental health. With acute psychiatric units at every district general hospital, and efforts being made to get the mentally sick well enough to stay in the community, the health centre will also have to be a place to which psychiatric patients readily turn.

What remains to be brought into the health centre and the orbit of the primary care doctor is all that has hitherto been the province of the local authority—the public health clinics for maternal and child welfare, for children's dental and general care and for dealing with some cases of mental deficiency. All the medical services of this nature must now be brought into health centres, and those existing clinics which are large enough or can be enlarged should rapidly be converted into health centres, retaining their old medical functions, now integrated with the rest of the NHS. One result will be changes in the care of the infant and the child, and a number of points will arise. We must continue those aspects of child care, especially school child care, which have been concerned with children in the mass. The observation of children at school has given us a mass of statistics about how our children are growing, and how their general health compares not only with earlier generations but with that of children in different parts of the country. We must also continue that very useful service which has permitted and enabled the school teacher to take action on noticing some sign of ill health in a pupil. Sometimes it is a sign not noted at home; and sometimes it is something that starts after the child has left home for school.

The family doctor will, of course, be seeing the children on his list, but we must not allow it to be thought that the special services for children should not continue, as part of the health centre. Dr A. L. Jacobs in the 1972 Somerville Hastings Memorial Lecture at Ruskin College declared: 'We must ensure that existing good child health services are not weakened by hasty and disruptive administrative changes'. His reason for saying this was that 'anyone familiar with a child health service under an advanced local authority will know it is a complex and comprehensive service which has to be run by a senior medical officer with special knowledge of child health and developmental paediatrics and requires a strong central organization and records'. The good parts of such a service must be retained and improved by the close collaboration of the G.P on the one hand and the hospital consultant paediatrician on the other.

There are three services that should be looked at again in an integrated service, and two of them at least should be fully brought into health centres: dentistry and sight testing. The third, pharmacy, is so intimately connected with the selling of all kinds of goods which have no connection with medicines that it may prove more difficult, but between health centres and hospitals a move must be made towards employing salaried pharmacists wherever possible. The hospital service already employs over 1,500 pharmacists and 1,200 pharmacy technicians, and in many hospital groups the Group Pharmacist plays an important part in the economic buying and use of drugs. This is another field in which geography imposes problems, and in most semi-rural areas it will be more economic and efficient to have a pharmacist at each health centre during the hours when most patients are being seen. With over 250 million prescriptions dispensed at a cost of over £150 million each year, this is a field in which organization and the closer working of pharmacist and doctor may produce savings. It must be remembered that one of the extras doctors get today is a fee for dispensing medicines in places where there is no chemist's shop. In a salaried service and in health centres, the £6 million spent on this each year will have to be used to build up a pharmacy service. One big result we may anticipate from a socially responsible health centre team is that as the health of the nation improves the prescribing of certain types of medicine will diminish. More than one-quarter of the drugs dispensed are given for their effects on the nervous system, and the health centre team, with closer links with the mental health service, may find it can do without some of the 70 million prescriptions written yearly.

The testing of eyes, the prescription of glasses and the dispensing of spectacles involves both doctors and trained opticians, and all three parts of the NHS. The dispensing opticians receive for their costs and their skill some £15 million a year. The testing of eyes is done by both doctors, the ophthalmic medical practitioners who get over £1.5 million, and the ophthalmic opticians, who are paid over £6 million a year. Between them they test nearly 6.5 million people each year. This is professional work which can very easily and with great advantage to patients be done at health centres. Clearly a decision has to be reached as to whether all sight testing should be in the hands of health centre opticians with the health centre physicians taking over, and very often referring to the hospital ophthalmic specialists, those cases in which disease other than simple optical defects are detected. In so far as opticians and the medical profession have not completely agreed on the division of eye work, close collaboration in the centres will be much better than the present division. There are already some hundreds of opticians working as salaried officers in the hospital service, and they will be united with the community opticians in one service.

Dentistry is an ideal service for inclusion in health centres and the experience already gained in this and other countries has proved that it is ideally organized as a salaried service. Great arguments have been produced by the medical profession as to why their clinical freedom must include freedom to prescribe, and British doctors are in this respect the most free in the world. But dentists have been given this clinical freedom only in salaried services, and it works equally well at a health centre in Scotland, a polyclinic in the USSR and a trade union clinic in San Francisco. Today the British dentist is controlled to a very large extent by the cost of every item of dental care which the dentist thinks is needed. There are nearly 11,000 dentists in England and Wales, and their average gross annual earnings are nearly £8,000 from the National Dental Service. But the way in which fees are fixed, the need to submit estimates for work to be done to the Dental Estimates Board, and the fact that as the patient is going to pay something and may be easily persuaded to pay more for particular items in order to avoid red tape, have all led to a situation in which this item of health care is very much in the market-place. In round figures the State pays about £60 million and the patients £15 million but dentists have to provide their own staff and equipment. It is claimed that in a form of service which uses a great variety of materials, and some expensive ones like gold, a degree of control of spending is necessary; but such a point arises only when we are thinking in terms of the market-place. In giving a service the socially responsible dentist should have the same freedom as the doctor to order a course of most expensive drugs if they are needed and to do so over a long period. There is no reason why a dentist who prescribes and supplies a gold inlay should be subject to other than the same kind of peer review, control by his own colleagues, as the doctor who for a chronic disease orders hundreds of pounds' worth of a life-saving drug. One big effect of bringing dentistry into the Health Centre would be that the public service could take steps to regularize and pay satisfactory salaries to trained dental technicians, and there could be a large increase in the numbers of dental hygienists and nurses.

It can now be seen why the health centre must become the focal point of all health activities in a district. The full team of what was envisaged as the most likely average size—six practitioners serving 15,000 people with the necessary receptionists and secretaries, the dentist, optician and pharmacist and their staff, the nurses and health visitors, the attached social workers, all add up to a substantial unit. There must be a considerable variation in size and staff so that local needs may be adequately served. The estimate of seventy for the total number of staff given in an early article on the subject, 'Get the Health Centres Going Now' (*Medicine Today and Tomorrow*, 1951), seems still to be reasonable. Since the health centre service discussed in 1951 is still relevant today, and will be during the next decade, it is summarized at the end of this chapter.

The buildings and the staff must also provide for educational activities including public film shows and lectures on specific subjects. But as we build new towns and rebuild old, the health centre should be more than the focal point on health. By its relationship with other healthful activities, recreational and educational, it should play its part in the overall improvement in the environment. Men once looked to temples as such focal points, and indeed the physician was intimately connected with such places. If man is to survive, the end of the twentieth century must make health the visible sign of his advancement, and man's comprehensive service for the maintenance of health the foundation on which it is ensured.

WHAT A HEALTH CENTRE WILL PROVIDE (1951)

If a health centre is to play its part in providing all that is implied by a 'comprehensive National Health Service available to every citizen,' its service should include or provide for the following:

1. Periodic examination for the maintenance of health and the early detection of disease.
2. A family doctor service organized from the Centre. Patients who are able will visit their family doctor at the centre; those who need home visits will arrange through the health centre for their family doctor to call. An appointment system, records, clerical and telephone assistance will be necessary for this purpose.
3. A twenty-four-hour emergency service.
4. The work done at present day health centres and clinics,

ante- and post-natal care, infant welfare, immunization, welfare officer, home nursing, etc.

5. A complete general dental service.
6. A general ophthalmic service.
7. A pharmaceutical service for NHS patients and internal supplies.
8. Health education and propaganda, and research
9. Special clinics, for example foot clinic or others which experience shows to be necessary.
10. The organization of factory health and accident services.
11. Rehabilitation and physiotherapy during convalescence.
12. Consultant services.

As medical science develops new functions may be added, and the administration of health centres must be elastic to allow this to happen. (An example which may call for early realization is that part of the compulsory post-graduation/pre-registration training of a young doctor may be at a health centre. The education of other health workers, particularly those with specific social duties, may also be completed by a period of health centre work.)

Chapter 19

Democratic Control

In another thirty years what will our hospitals be like? Are the new ones now being built so different from the old that we need take only a few more steps in alteration for the future buildings and functions to bear no resemblance to the late nineteenth-century places now being pulled down? Our ancestors built in the old workhouses which led to the poor-law hospitals such similar and typical buildings that today they are still recognizable. This generation is putting up hospital blocks of the same style as the office towers of every city, and they are likely to be there in a hundred years, causing the same problems of replacement. There are a host of debatable points in what is now the best plan we have, because it has not been built to fulfil an ideological plan as to what our hospital patients need. It can, of course, be argued that since the average hospital stay is now only a few days the architecture and decor are not so important. But even for a short stay, amenities are important; and in any case we must ask how much better are we planning for the long-stay cases and, above all, for the aged. Why do we still refuse to build our hospitals for the nation entirely of single rooms if, as the wealthy claim, private pay beds should be in single rooms and should have individual toilets, telephones and television? Single-room hospitals are much easier, and therefore cheaper, to run than hospitals with large wards, and are much more comfortable. But the matter is still discussed with a strong class bias, untested—that the middle class like single rooms, and the less affluent like to be herded together with little or no privacy. If AD 2,000 is to have anything different in real terms we ought to be planning something different now.

We have said less about hospitals than about primary health care in our blueprint so far because they are fundamentally technological institutions in which humanity must be served, but in which certain scientific principles must have priority. This is especially so in surgical wards of all kinds. The techniques of modern surgery, and the accompanying anaesthetics, are almost fantastic in comparison with what early surgeons could even try to do. The improvements have been made possible by ways of avoiding the great threats the surgeon has to face, such as infection of wounds, loss of blood and upsets of the whole body chemistry. The great assistance the surgeon has had from the bacteriologist, the blood transfusion experts and the biochemist have made much of modern surgery safe. Other technical experts have had to help, and they have come from many branches of industry, but basically it has been the growth of hospital laboratories and the attention given by doctors trained in scientific methods that have made it possible for the expert and experienced surgeons to achieve their best results. Sterilization of materials, guarding against the entry of dangerous germs, and perfecting of techniques to treat infections with antibiotics, have also reduced the risk of bacterial invasion. One part of this, the building up of Central Sterile Supply Departments to supply all materials used in operating theatres, casualty departments and wards in a sterile condition, has done much to aid the surgeon and has, as mentioned earlier, made modifications in buildings possible. On biochemistry and blood transfusion we need not dwell further, for what they mean today has been repeatedly recorded.

Hospital care is episodic and no one would want it to be more than that, yet in the context of a district general hospital the hospital staff must move into a much more continuous relation with the community and with the doctors and health workers outside the hospital. This we have discussed earlier, but now as we try to prepare an administrative blueprint we have to ask what part the hospital staffs, and especially the doctors who, up to the moment, have often had a leading role in the work of hospital management committees, are to play in health district administration. Are they to retain, and possibly increase, the executive duties they have had, or to be advisers only in the part of the service in which they work? Lay committees and lay executive officers will wish to have advice from their own medical and other health workers and that we can discuss as a separate subject. But are we to retain the principle, which had to be fought for, that an officer of the NHS can also be a member of its controlling bodies? In an SMA document *Administration of the Health Service* published in 1951 the proposition was made (and has been in effect since then) that as a matter of principle, 'it must be established that a doctor is also a citizen. This seemingly self-evident proposition is revolutionary. It means that, as a citizen, the doctor can sit on the authority responsible for the service in which he is employed.' The article went on to say that this 'is one of the points which distinguish a socialized health service from other forms of State medicine.' This is the starting point for any discussion on the NHS of AD 2,000 if one believes that, at the rate of change we now see in our institutions, socialization of services must be one of the aims of society. We shall take it as part of the aim of this blueprint. The position of officers in a service is one part of the story, the other being the participation of the citizens, in health and in sickness.

But there are one or two further points about hospitals as institutions that must be considered. We shall assume that plans for district general hospitals, of which we believe the ideal size is about 1,000 beds, will mature, and that building will go ahead rapidly. But not even the latest promises to spend more money on building will catch up with the need in the next twenty years. Much more money will be needed if all the necessary new buildings are to be provided. It must be remembered that the district health unit will have its satellites and these will be of varied types. It is probably in smaller units, less elaborately built and equipped, that much of the care of the aged can be arranged. But these should be, generally, new units, purpose built, for there is nothing less suitable for the aged (or for any other disabled group) than the older type of building, the cottage hospital with wings added at different levels, the former poor-law building which in spite of interior vamping remains gaunt and uninviting. These must be replaced. It is unlikely, if we leave this to regional or even area bodies, that people will care enough to force the changes. The people in a district, the future inhabitants of these buildings, are the people to make a habitable and pleasurable set of buildings for their own aged friends.

The district must also be stressed as the area from within which the district general hospital cannot refuse to assist any citizen. We do not want boundaries, but we do need hospitals and hospital staffs who feel they have a responsibility. For acute care the Emergency Bed Service is essential; but even when it operates effectively, it must still be made clear, as is not always the case today, that a citizen seeking medical aid must be given it. That aid should be the best we can organize, and *Health Trends* (February 1972) had a most significant point to make in an editorial on manpower. Having indicated that hospital medical staff increased by more than 880 between 1 October 1970 and 30 September 1971, it went on: 'However it is regrettable that less than one-third of the increase was in the consultant grade'. The editorial continued: 'There has been no improvement in the number of those first appointed to the consultant grade and no reduction in the average age on appointment'. It is imperative that the number of consultants goes up, but it would also be of great help, and a possible inspiration, if younger men could be brought in with newer ideas. The profession should not need to be told by anyone else that if it is a consultant's duty to see all the cases at his clinic he must see them, but he will do this automatically when his education stresses social responsibility, and private practice does not enter into his calculations as to the time he must spend in his hospital.

What the nation wants to buy, then, is a hospital service adequate to the point where beds are waiting for patients and the so-called waiting list is no more than an administrative device to smooth out the work load, and is not an excuse for delays; a service which is adequately staffed and equipped to do a modern job. It must not only be comprehensive, it must be efficient and it must be humane. It should be as free from errors as is humanly possible, but it should have built in safeguards and checks, even an ombudsman. It must be flexible, and its aim must be tomorrow while it deals with today economically but with decision. It must try to find the solution to the problem of co-operation between highly trained health workers, the suppliers, and the citizens, the consumers of health care. In finding a way to treat all the sick and to do so in a socialized service, a lead can be given that may be an example in many other fields.

A comprehensive service for 55 million people is a large undertaking. We have yet to discuss what it will cost, and in doing so we have all the incalculables of future inflation, but we can say that in another twenty years the service will still have half a million hospital beds, many more than one million workers, and will need from the national income not less than £3,000 million. Such an undertaking needs an administration machine but one that is unique, because it cannot be priced in any way that will show how much profit it makes. It must be judged indirectly on the way deaths and morbidity from certain diseases are changing, by the number of people living well after the traditional seventy years, and so on. It must be as efficient in a managerial sense as we can make it. Its administration must be as efficient as democracy permits—for democracy always carries risks of inefficiency which must be accepted if our democracy is to mean anything. It must have an administration responsive and responsible to the people and their needs, and it must be managerially sound since it is accountable to Government and Parliament. As we approach AD 2,000 it must become socialized, a great co-operative effort to take a healthy nation in a healthy environment into the unforeseeable possibilities of the next hundred years.

So we must begin once more with the ordinary citizen. What does democracy in the context of the control of a social service mean? Professor Peter Townsend writing of all the social services (*The Lancet*, 5 Spetember 1970) said: 'The public and the consumer must be involved more frequently than at present in the management of the social services (whether schools, residential homes, hospitals or day centres)'. Ultimately it may be that one chain of responsible bodies will deal with both health and social services, as the central Department of Health and Social Services implies, but the dividing line should be between those items which are of a service nature, financed centrally, and those for which people have paid contributions. The criterion for getting the latter is financial need and is strictly on an insurance principle; the former are a right of the citizen. For the moment, however, we have to think of administering the health services and creating any necessary co-ordinating machinery between health and social services.

Administration in health need have only three levels. Ministerial documents have in recent times suggested two or three tiers and a document circulated in February 1972 by the DHSS, but not yet published, suggested four levels of management. We believe that three are necessary and enough, but their size, distribution and membership are vital. The lowest level is the most controversial and if it is not right the rest may well be wrong.

At the lowest level the citizen must be able to understand and to influence this service, the quality of which sooner or later may be a matter of life or death to him or his family. The administrative size should therefore, subject to efficiency, be small enough for him to be aware of its ramifications and to feel he can genuinely voice an opinion about it. He can do that best by voting for the members of the controlling committee. The committee must itself have a large enough job to do, and power to make variations and changes, must have some control over finance, and its members should be elected from the people. Democracy has been defined in many ways but the British basic principle remains, that public services run for and financed by the public can be controlled democratically only by an elected body. To argue that this may not throw up people with 'managerial skill' is to mistake what management means and to deny our democratic principles. When election produces members who do not appear competent the electorate has to make the necessary change.

In all electoral matters the one question to be decided is the size of the unit. Discussions so far on some kind of area committee have been quite unrealistic and vague; and the areas are exceedingly variable because they have nothing to do with health care needs but with a desire to have the health unit coterminous with the local authorities. Thus the areas proposed vary from some twenty with 200,000 people to some ten or twelve with nearly 2,000,000.

If however our discussions on the size of the area served by one district general hospital, with between ten and twenty health centres drawing their special consultant and specialist services they need from that hospital and its laboratories etc., are valid – and we believe they are – then here is the ideal basic 'brick' from which to build a good three-tier administrative structure. We would have in each of such districts, of which there would be about 200 for the whole country (some considerations might necessitate a few being as large as 300,000 people, but never larger), a district health committee of, say, fifteen elected members, who would appoint their own chairman. They would control and administer all the health functions of their district.

Management would be in the hands of their officers, some of whom might, to answer the legal position of being agents of the Secretary of State, be appointed by the middle tier, the regional health authority. The district health committee (DHC) would prepare its own budget and from the money made available would have full responsibility for all decisions on the day-to-day running of all the health facilities in its district. It would be expected to create the necessary liaison with the Director of Social Services, his staff and his controlling authority. It would be advised by various advisory bodies largely drawn from the health workers of hospital and health service. Doctors and all health workers who wished, independently or as members of a political party, to stand for election to the DHC, would be free to do so.

While the district health committee must have the task of planning its own services, these must fit into the national plan and major building projects, for which the money comes from the capital budget, may have to be agreed at the centre. However the real planning of the services must be on a regional basis, for two reasons: the service is not to be run from Whitehall (or the Elephant and Castle, where the Department of Health is now housed), hence an intermediate planning authority is necessary; and the hospital service, even when the whole of the health facilities are integrated, needs a considerable degree of regional planning. In some specialities the resources available need to be planned to avoid duplication, and also to ensure that very special units are given enough money and that the area they serve is well defined. Experience of the regional hospital boards has shown that our present regions are about the right number and size and certainly cannot be any larger if they are to have any kind of control over the periphery. Special interests like undergraduate and postgraduate training, the appointment of some if not all specialists, the fostering and funding of research, special problems that go beyond the ordinary budget of the district general hospital, all these and more need the attention of a regional health authority (RHA).

At this level, at which popular election might be a little difficult and not very well supported, the RHA need not be elected, but should for various reasons be representational. Those who know their health service history will be aware of various attempts in the past twenty years to develop a proper relationship between the regional hospital board and some of its hospital management committees. RHB members were asked to serve on an HMC but the liaison was never perfected.

With between ten and fifteen district health committees in each region in England and Wales (Scotland has already decided on a slightly different method), the first group who must be represented on the RHA are the district committees. Approximately half of the members of the RHA should come from below, thus ensuring that through their elected representatives at the lower level the people's voice would be heard and the districts would act in unison. One or two members would therefore come to the RHA from each of the districts. The rest of the members would be appointed by the Secretary of State, but some interests must be represented. First the Department of Health must appoint three or four members, who might be officers or lay people with knowledge and skill in administration. Other interests – the major trade unions, the universities, the medical profession and other health workers, the local authorities – might all be asked to nominate a representative to the RHA. The formula should be binding so that the interests named would be sure of a place. It was a fault in the 1946 Act that while such bodies had a right to nominate they had no guarantee that their nominee would be appointed.

Such a regional health authority would correct many of the faults in the regional hospital board system. It would create a true meeting-place of all the interested parties, and the national strategy for health, pronounced by the Secretary of State, would be discussed by the framers of that policy, the planners of the service and those responsible for seeing that the service fulfilled the plan in a way that was never possible in the RHB/HMC set-up. It would also be a meeting-place for producers and consumers of health care with enough people, the special representatives, acting in both capacities. All three levels would now be very clearly administrative bodies, making plans and policy decisions and leaving the way clear for the straight managerial functions of the appointed officers to be carried out effectively. Sir Keith Joseph's often expressed desire for greater managerial skill in the NHS has been translated by many of the statements made by other people into an attempt to hand both administration and management to one group of officers acting independently of public control. It is time the issue was clarified. Managers of the highest technical skill are needed throughout the NHS. They must be appointed to do a particular job, managing the staffs, managing the kitchens, the transport, the supplies and so on, and they must be backed up by first-class financial management.

Administration, on the other hand, involves both committee members and those officers whose primary duties include formulating new plans, dealing with problems as they arise: but it involves more than the one discipline or group which a manager can deal with, and above all advising the statutory committees on all matters requiring decisions and involving strategy. Both managerial and administrative staffs should be as low in numbers as is compatible with efficiency. A document issued to various parts of the service by the DHSS on this subject confuses administration with management, suggesting a four-tier system of managers. This would have led to an enormous increase in the health service bureaucracy without a single extra patient being treated. Whenever a proposal like this semi-secret document is made, it must be judged by how many more patients would benefit from it and by what amount the standard of care would be raised.

There are two further questions about the RHA members which need fresh thinking. On the question of the chairman of such a body there appear to be only two alternatives, that he is appointed by the Secretary of State, or that he is elected by the members. The chairman of the RHBs had to give a lot of time to the work; the chairman in an integrated service will have to give more. So he might require to be paid more than expenses, more even than enough to compensate him for loss of earnings, and it seems logical that the Secretary of State should seek out and appoint the best man he can find. The danger is that this is then looked on as a managerial appointment, whereas the chairman of such a body must never exercise managerial authority. His duty is as controller of the policy-making administrative machine, and he must be prepared to speak out for his RHA when necessary against government decisions. If democracy is our aim he should be chosen and appointed by the RHA knowing the size of job he is taking on, and on the understanding that he will be recompensed for the time he gives to it.

It would also appear necessary for more generosity to be shown to the members of both RHAs and DHCs than has been the case in the past with hospital committee members. Above all, compensation for loss of earnings must be made to enable ordinary people to give time to their duties, for it will not be only a question of an occasional meeting. Hospitals, health centres and so on will have to be visited and time spent on seeking the views of patients and joining in the educational work that is so necessary. We have spoken of education on health; but the public also need education on the service, on what is available and on how it is provided, so that all can take an interest. There must be no false modesty about this question of payment for doing a public duty. The days of the village squire and the town mayor running a voluntary hospital have gone. We move into a socialized health service in which administrative ability and public interest must be the criteria for election.

If we now look at Figure 19.1, we see that the simplest part of the administrative machine is the committee structure, with national strategy at the centre, regional planning and district provision. It will be the supporting, advisory structure that will complicate the picture. How much advice will the two levels need? Should it come from the local or regional staffs or from specially appointed committees? What medical advice and administration should each level have? Can a joint health workers' committee be constituted today or must we wait for the development of a more communal spirit than exists at present? It is often much easier for staff groups to give a purely technical opinion than a wide-ranging view of the needs of the community. Where does medical administration come in? In the regional hospital boards and hospital management committees the senior control was shared by the senior lay, medical, nursing and finance officers. Then the Cogwheel system was tried, a form of medical executive constituted of one member of each specialty, the chairman of a specialty committee if there were enough specialists to form a committee; while the medical administrator faded out or resigned. No one finds that this system works at all well. It was an attempt to involve as many of the hospital medical staff as possible in administration, and in some way to introduce a note of democracy into the medical staff committees which had established themselves at the start of the NHS with a variety of constitutions.

Now the Secretary of State calls for better managerial skills, the position of medical administrators must be considered in greater depth than ever before and fairly quick decisions must be made. The Cogwheel report (*Organization of Medical Work in Hospitals*, 1967) abolished the position of individual medical superintendent but did

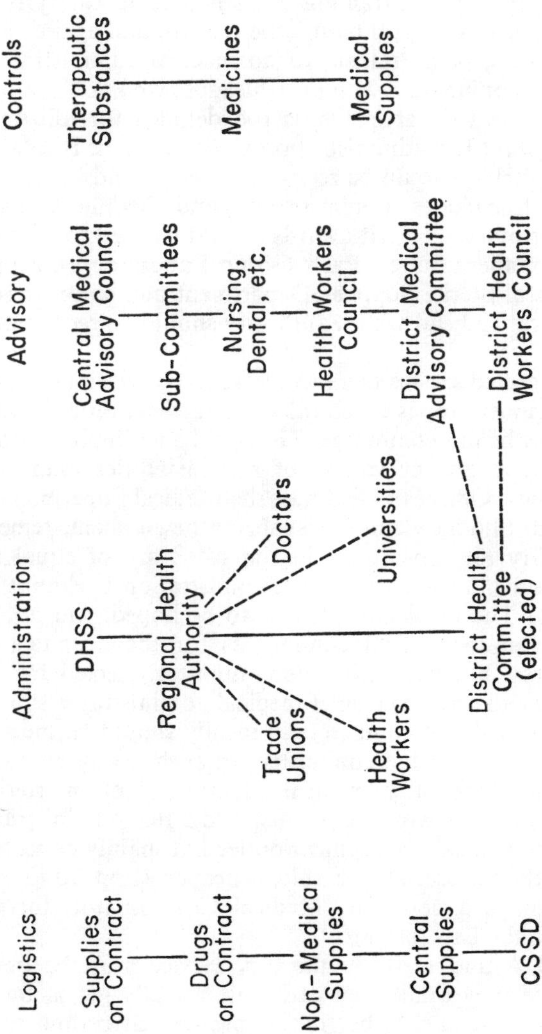
Logistics
Supplies on Contract
Drugs on Contract
Non-Medical Supplies
Central Supplies
CSSD
Administration
DHSS
Regional Health Authority
Trade Unions
Health Workers
Doctors
Universities
District Health Committee (elected)
Advisory
Central Medical Advisory Council
Sub-Committees
Nursing, Dental, etc.
Health Workers Council
District Medical Advisory Committee
District Health Workers Council
Controls
Therapeutic Substances
Medicines
Medical Supplies

Figure 19.1

not abolish the work the superintendent did. That work was to be taken over by a 'small medical executive committee'; the chairman of that committee was to become the medical administrator for five years, and to get special training in his new temporary job.

In a book of this general nature the case for and against a medical man who elects, or is trained, to do medical administration for a whole unit in conjunction with his colleagues who do the administration of their own departments, is too detailed for full discussion. Every consultant has administration to do and if it is a fairly large part of his work it should be recognized: he should be appointed to a post which includes administration and the money at present secretly distributed as merit awards should be used to provide extra payments for these duties. Each Group Laboratory, Group X-ray, Group Central Sterile Supplies Department and so on should have an administrative head whose authority should be recognized in the salary structure.

In an integrated service there will have to be decisions about which medical administrator is to be the chief medical officer and adviser to the district health committee. This will be an important post, and will have much greater variety of responsibilities than either the former Medical Officer of Health or the Medical Superintendent of a hospital had. Should we now visualize a new system, remembering that in theory all consultants in the NHS are of equal standing clinically, and that whatever the administration it cannot be truly hierarchical? The medical staff, it is to be hoped, will not think in terms of separate medical committees for the hospitals and the health centres, but will have one committee, elected from all the doctors in the district. The chief medical administrator should never be chairman of that committee and ideally should be the secretary, that is the servant of the committee. In such a way we can depart from the old idea of a medical superintendent interfering with every other doctor's work, and substitute a real administrator, with some routine clinical or technical duties but mainly concerned with seeing that the service, as available, is properly applied to every sick person. Perhaps a new title, Medical Co-ordinator, for example, would make the issue clearer.

Every RHA and DHC in the new service must be free to ask advice where they think they can most usefully get it, but equally the doctors must always be free to proffer advice and must have access to the official bodies. At RHA level there will automatically be doctors who are members, and they may present the staff views and ideas. At DHC level it is still necessary to consider whether this elected committee should co-opt extra members, and if so whether they should represent doctors and other health workers as two groups or one. We are still in a transitional stage towards socialization when such distinctions will have no operative value, and in a transition a compromise, to retain separate doctors' representations, may be necessary. If so, then all other health workers, probably through health workers councils, should select members for co-option or any other form of representation. Every effort, however, should be made to reduce the number of committees and the time spent in meetings, and much will depend on the quality of officers which the integrated service attracts.

Ultimately, we would hope within a decade, each district should have its health workers council on which everyone employed is represented. Integrated views can then be given, for all groups will find that they can reach agreement more quickly when they meet as one. The same must apply to trade unions. Health workers are joining unions in far greater numbers and we must reach the position of having only one trade union to represent all health workers. On the medical side it is regrettable that much of the trade union work, negotiating on terms of service, has been done by the BMA, which by its own rules is prohibited from being a trade union and so could never take the essential step of affiliating to the TUC. It should revert to its original function as a professional and scientific association, or it should change its rules and become a trade union when it might lead the struggle to unite all health workers. The Soviet Union has a single Medical Workers Union which appears to increase the spirit of team-work in every health group, and makes the whole question of advisory committees very much simpler.

Because the NHS is only twenty-four years old we still spend too much time debating what has to be done and how it should be done. When we manage to understand that an integrated service has the single aim of doing everything for health and doing it at the highest possible standard, the arguments should die down. When agreement has been reached on the amount of money the NHS is to have, if it is adequate a great deal of discussion that now takes place will be unnecessary. When a proper managerial system is worked out it must be coupled with departmental budgets and the manager of a department, whether medical or professional, must be free to operate within the budget. Democracy, however, will insist that even then the staff of a department must have the opportunity to meet over purely departmental matters, and it is from such staff committees that the health workers council should be built up. An attempt to show the routes of contact is given in Figure 19.2.

As the next decade comes to an end how much will human beings be dealing with health and how much will computers have taken over? There are ecologists who advocate that we have to curb machines, not destroy them like Luddites, but control them socially, in order to employ the millions who might otherwise be unemployed. Certainly in a health service human beings, consumers and producers of health care, must be superior to hardware, and a health service should never do anything which increases the amount of waste material that has to be disposed of, and is sometimes almost indestructible. One of the biggest errors in this field has been the

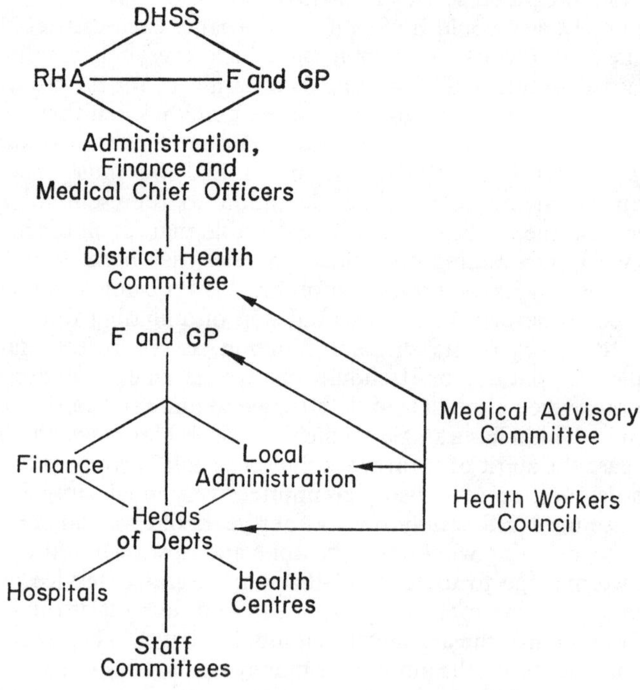

Figure 19.2

acceptance by the Department of Health of the manufacturers advocacy of disposable syringes and needles, plastic blood bags, plastic bottles and commercially manufactured sterile supplies generally. To take an example which is well documented, many hospitals had built up excellent services for the supply of sterile syringes, using glass syringes. A system like the present author's Kingston Syringe box was cheap and efficient, used human beings instead of plastic, and produced no waste. The DHSS has made contracts with manufacturers to supply 10 million plastic syringes, much inferior to glass in the hands of the doctor, and all of them have to be disposed of by fire. The example can be multiplied. Man has to take a close look at everything he does to see how it will affect the environment and people. By reversing the move to use commercially prepared plastic materials (discardable but hardly disposable) and using materials producing less waste and employing people presently unemployed the NHS could save money and set an example of social responsibility.

Computers will, naturally, play an increasing part in the recording and collating of clinical material. One of the very first advantages that was expected to arise from a national service was that a double picture would be built up, that of the individual through a running record of clinical observation in which GPs and hospital records would be brought together, and that of the health of the whole community. Both tasks have been started and by the end of the decade should be normal practice. By then people will have lost the fear that such records will in some way lessen confidentiality in doctors' findings, and will realise that accuracy and ready availability in precise information about one's previous medical history can be of life-saving importance. With increasing health education people will understand that the old idea of secrecy, which some doctors carried to the point (an illegal one) of not telling patients about their own blood test results, or not showing them X-ray plates of their own body, is neither valid nor necessary. What the computer records about an individual's body must clearly belong to the individual and not to the doctor or the State, but he should be happy that the record is there and is being used for scientific purposes.

By AD 2,000 man may have acquired much greater skill in maintaining life, a greater ability to keep bodies alive with artificial machines, hearts and heart valves and pace-makers, kidney dialysis in a more simple personal form, more delicate control of biochemical functions and the preservation of blood and other tissues for long periods. It is very unlikely that he will be able to transplant a brain, but he may transplant most other organs with a high, but still incomplete, degree of success. Will he have settled the ethical problems that all these advances raise and will he have saved the human race by a drastic cutting down of the birth rate? And at the other end of the life span will he have not only agreed to but made possible simple voluntary euthanasia for the disabled aged? Let us hope that man will have taken world medicine out of the market-place and, by following Britain's great humanist lead, will have provided a system for health care that will start the next century on an optimistic note.

Chapter 20

Cost and Ethics

How, it may be asked, are cost and ethics joined together? Is not the question of how much money is to be spent a political and economic matter? And are not ethics the philosophical basis on which man and his society behave and interact? That would certainly have been true in the hundred years before 1948. It is only partly true today even in health, and in trying to visualize the health care system for AD 2,000 we must believe that society will have moved into a new era, one in which no political or economic decisions are made without the full ethical inferences having been drawn and acted upon. We are dealing with one of the most important aspects of human welfare and, as Titmuss has remarked, 'Human welfare is an ethical concept'. That being so, health care must be taken completely out of the ordinary commercial atmosphere if it is to be the altruistic service it must be. True, all the workers in the service will be earning their living from the work they do. Nevertheless they will be giving the whole of their time, without the complexities of trying to do private practice as well, and will be serving their patients with a dedication which will very often attain the highest spirit of altruism. This is the kind of altruism which Titmuss goes on to discuss in *The Gift Relationship* as touching 'every aspect of life and affecting the whole fabric of values'. There is no way in which we can calculate the money value of saving lives, but we can value the spirit in which it is done. Health care loses its value as a unifying force in a community if it is not based on firm ethical decisions. Once society has decided on that question, society must then look at the cost of the service in a very different light and must be prepared to spend as much as the service needs.

As figures in earlier chapters showed we have not spent in Britain as high a proportion of our gross national product on health as we should have done, and the slow rise to today's approximate figure of 5 per cent would have been much more rapid if the ethical principles had been wholly acceptable to the governments we had between 1951 and 1964. Between 1950 and 1955 there was indeed a fall in the amount of money made available for health, from 4.07 to 3.40 per cent of the GNP. The subsequent rise was very slow; even after 1964 the rate of increase was too small, and after that date the most rapid increase was in capital expenditure. The whole picture is made more intricate by the continuous inflation of these years and quite a high proportion of any increase is taken up by the rising population, above all by the necessary extra care for the aged. As we have seen, all countries are having to spend more and Britain must now make a decision which can be sustained for the next twenty years.

One difficulty is that no government in the past twenty years appears to have reached a figure for annual spending by any rational consideration of priorities. It may be that a rational system cannot be achieved while we spend as much as we do on defence, but we must change the present position. Nicholas Bosanquet (*Labour and Inequality*, 1972) says that 'the overall spending decision in health does not emerge from any coherent framework of choice between competing projects'. It might be easier to reach such a decision if 'the output to be obtained from extra spending was clearly measurable', but that is not entirely the case. All past experience shows that when extra money is spent in an organized service (but not in a free enterprise system), greater output, greater benefits to the individual and to the nation's health record can be attained; but it is not susceptible to ordinary cost-benefit auditing. One factor has to some extent worked against the NHS getting more money, its own success. It is difficult to rouse public opinion to make strong demands when the service is doing a good job and is completely accepted by the nation. Bosanquet points out that 'within the NHS some pressures operate to push up spending on the acutely ill. But spending on the chronic sick, the mentally ill and handicapped has few powerful advocates'. We must reach the point when no underprivileged group needs to have advocates. It is the task of the health service administrators to identify groups who are not getting adequate service, to attend to the still considerable variations between one part of the country and another, and to see that resources are evenly distributed. The NHS has also to learn to use its manpower to the greatest advantage, to discover what are the best sizes of units for different purposes, and to look at the relationships, most of them historic rather than planned, between workers with differing skills and responsibilities. Training must however be coupled with better promotion prospects, and all workers must be made to feel they are making a worthwhile contribution to the service.

The cost of the NHS each year has so far been calculated by

making each unit work out its annual budget, which is then scrutinized, and usually cut, by succeeding stages of authority up to the Chancellor of the Exchequer. Budgeting is a worthwhile exercise if departments are to be kept actively watching their spending. But the nation should make the decision as to how much is needed overall and budgets should be as readily adjusted upwards as downwards by the Department, the RHA and the DHC before they finally come back to the administrator who made the initial calculations. We are not spending per capita anything like the USA, Sweden or the USSR; given the extra, say up to 6 per cent of the GNP, not only could existing services be made to give the highest quality of care, they could be persuaded to initiate future developments and look far beyond the present. Six per cent would still leave the UK with the most economical of health services, for those countries which do not appear to spend as much do not give a comprehensive service or do not give a universal service, and do not give a service free at the time of use. The present charges can be abolished and the whole service restored to its intended basis.

The 6 per cent, however, is needed for current daily expenditure; capital for new buildings and especially to hasten the provision of health centres and get well beyond the promised 500 by 1974, should be accounted separately. It is time the NHS accounts included some estimate of the capital cost of the service and some indication of how quickly our assets depreciate. Every hospital department which needs new equipment has to fight for it without reference to what the old equipment cost and what, in ordinary financing terms, its written-down value is (X-ray is an exception). The fact that the service given to the patient is not to be charged or regarded on ordinary commercial lines is no reason why sound financial principles should not apply to buildings and equipment. None of our big monopoly capitalist firms would fail to know how much capital had been invested in land, buildings, transport and so on, or to have calculations made as to how long it could be expected to last. The NHS manages without knowing either factor.

How do we collect and apply 6 per cent of our GNP? At present approximately 85 per cent of the money available comes from public funds, taxation and rates, and 10 per cent from insurance contributions. No plan that has been suggested – more payments for services, charges for every stay in hospital, extra contributions from employers – is any more than a device to move part of the cost from one section of society to another; and the move so far has been more a move from the relatively poor to the rich than the other way round. Economists may argue such devices in great detail, but they have no place in discussion once the ethical and political decisions to have a universal service have been made. Indeed as soon as the new integrated service comes into being the part of the cost now borne by the rates will have to come from central funds; and the insurance contributions, which have nothing to do with who gets the service, are simply another form of taxation (which costs money and manpower to collect). A universal system must be financed from central taxation. There is no form of insurance, sick fund, mutual or profit-making in any country which has proved capable of financing a comprehensive service for all, and no new evidence on the subject is forthcoming for more and more governments are having to step in and subsidize or supply essential services. By the end of 1972 more than half the spending on services in the USA, the bulwark of insurance programmes, will be provided by governmental funds, and any country which now tries to avoid changing from health insurance to a health service will be defeated by the continually increasing cost of and demand for health care.

We have quoted many witnesses to the strength of these arguments and could find many more. We have given many reasons why Sir Keith Joseph was justified in saying of the service he, a Conservative, controls, that 'the standards of specialist, general practice and community medicine are probably higher than in any other country in the world'; and we have tried to confirm that by personal study and visits to more than twenty countries and hundreds of health facilities. We have tried to show that the ethical basis of the British National Health Service is the only correct one for a personal service dealing with fitness to live and the ability of the individual to stand up to our modern environment. We have discussed some faults and deficiencies, none of which are inherent in a national service of this kind, but which arise from lack of sufficient money or staff and from faulty ideas among health workers who have not had a chance to assist in administration or have not developed the essential sense of social responsibility.

The specification written between 1940 and 1945 at least settled principles. There was less doubt about which form of health care was being bought than about how much the nation would have to pay. In attempting a new plan there is still much to be specified as to what will be provided and still doubt as to how much will have to be paid. It is clear that if a genuine attempt is made to have a comprehensive service for all citizens, and to give all the same high standard of care, the price will still rise; but economies can be achieved by better organization. That organization must employ good managerial staff, but the policy control must be shared by good administrators, including medical men and women, and representatives of the people, of the patients as citizens. A plan is therefore put forward for a three-tier system—the Department of Health and Social Security taking control of the national strategy for health; regional health authorities in charge of planning and consisting of representatives from the Department, and the lower tier, which should be an elected District Health Committee. The latter should cover a population usually under 250,000 and should be responsible for all the health services and interests in its own district.

The two outstanding needs of the next decade are the provision of health centres giving full general services, medical, dental, optical and pharmaceutical, through the agency of salaried officers; and the setting up of an Occupational Health Service which should be closely linked with the health centre service. Some 500 health centres are promised by 1974; the full chain of 2,000 should be built before 1980 if medicine is to become a true social service before the end of the century. The hospitals must be of every necessary type, including day and night facilities, the staffs should be full-time officers, and private practice should no longer be permitted inside the NHS. The whole staff of the NHS should participate in control and development through health workers councils; but medical administration, backed by medical advisory committees, should be put on a proper managerial footing. New promotional and salary ladders should be devised and free movement and training between grades encouraged.

Finally the public should be educated both about the health service and about health. Vigorous propaganda to deal with recognized problems, such as cigarette smoking in the individual, prevention of disease as by fluoridation of water, active intervention whenever the environment is threatened, birth control freely and simply advocated and encouraged, special problems of the aged, their care and, when society is ready for it, voluntary euthanasia – all these and many other matters must be part of the new plan. Health care must continue to be based on the primary care physician whose work should be recognized as a separate speciality, and he should give the inspiration in all matters of disease prevention. Mental health services should be developed in every way that can be shown to assist people to overcome the stress of the modern environment; and the permanently disabled, mentally or physically, accidental or genetic, should be given greater care. Machines, computers, automatic blood testing equipment and so on, should be used to give better care but not allowed to dominate a service in which human contact is the prime necessity. The health service must, by its own way of employing people, by the help it gives to employing the disabled, be an example to the rest of industry.

Meantime the nation should do many other things that concern health. Education must be improved and our schools should aim at turning out psychologically healthy students. Poverty, a prime cause of ill health, must be abolished, not so much by increasing industrialization as by better organization and equitable distribution of the nation's wealth. People should not become diseased because they have an inadequate diet, or if they are old suffer from cold, or work in a hostile environment. Mankind has a long way to go to theoretical perfection. Britain and its NHS should start the last quarter of this century determined to wipe out all preventable disease, to safeguard the environment and to realize the dream of a healthy nation.

Bibliography

There is a very large literature on many aspects of health care. An excellent summary of what a student of the subject might consult (over six hundred books and articles), is given by Battistella; and a monthly list of new publications is given in *Medical Care Review* (University of Michigan, Ann Arbor, US).

Abel-Smith, B. *An International Study of Health Expenditure*, Public Health Papers No 32, World Health Organization, Geneva, 1967.

Battistella, Roger M. *Health Care Organization*, AUPHA, Washington, DC, 1971.

Bryant, J. *Health and the Developing World*, Cornell University Press, 1969.

Dubos René *Man, Medicine and Environment*, F. A. Praeger, New York, 1968.

Evang, Karl *Health Service, Society and Medicine*, London University Press, 1968.

Evang, K., Murray, D. S., and Lear, W. J. *Medical Care and Family Security*, Prentice Hall, 1963.

Fry, John *Medicine in Three Societies*, Medical and Technical Publishing Company, 1969.

Fry, J., and Farndale, W. J. *International Medical Care*, Medical and Technical Publishing Company, 1972.

Lindsey, Almont *Socialized Medicine*, Chapel Hill, 1962.

Roemer, Milton I. *The Organization of Medical Care under Social Security*, International Labour Office, Geneva, 1969.

Titmuss, R. M. *The Gift Relationship*, George Allen & Unwin, 1971.

Townsend, P., and Bosanquet, N. *Labour and Inequality*, Fabian Society, 1972.

Index